*This book is dedicated to everyone in pain
in the hope that it will bring you relief.*

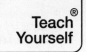
Teach®
Yourself

Beat Your Pain and Find Lasting Relief

Paul Jenner

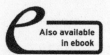

Also available in ebook

Meet the author

Paul Jenner is the author of more than 30 books, specializing in health, personal development and life skills, and has reported from all over the world. He believes in approaching pain relief from as many different directions as possible. There is often no single technique, he says, that will bring about complete relief. It's a combination of techniques that's needed. In addition to *Beat Your Pain and Find Lasting Relief*, his titles include *Beat Your Depression*, *How to be Happier*, *Transform Your Life With NLP* and *Help Yourself to Live Longer*. His books have been translated into several languages, including French, Spanish, Dutch, German and Chinese. He has written for national newspapers including the *Daily Telegraph* and *The Observer*. When not working he enjoys activities that promote a spiritual connection with landscape and nature, including hiking, mountain biking, snowboarding, swimming and sailing. He and his partner divide their time between England, France and Spain. He would be delighted to hear from you on his website.

www.pauljenner.eu

Acknowledgements

A very special thank you to Victoria Roddam, my editor at Hodder & Stoughton.

Contents

Introduction

This book is something of a prequel to a book I wrote called *How to be Happier*. Some people were telling me they couldn't even think of implementing the ideas in that book because they were in too much pain. They needed to get rid of the pain first. So I decided to write something for them.

I discovered that there's an enormous amount of pain in the world. According to various studies, around one-fifth of the world's population suffers chronic pain, with women more affected than men, and the figure rises to one-third among the elderly. And, of course, everyone suffers acute pain from time to time.

I also discovered that at least one-third of sufferers are dissatisfied with the medical treatment they're receiving for their pain, and the figure could be much higher – in one online survey 78 per cent of respondents said they were dissatisfied.

So the principal aim of this book is to put you in charge of your own pain reduction programme. I do that by focusing on the things you can do yourself. So, for example, I haven't included hypnosis but I have included self-hypnosis. I haven't included physiotherapy but I have included physical exercises, as well as self-treatment with transcutaneous electrical nerve stimulation (TENS) and ultrasound. The main exceptions to this concept of self-treatment are prescribed painkillers, a huge range of which are described in Chapter 2, massage (although self-massage is included) and acupuncture, because it's become such a popular self-prescribed remedy.

I'm conscious of the fact that many of you will have been in pain for some time and will already have tried various treatments. But if you find just one therapy in this book that's useful and new to you then it will have been worthwhile. Hopefully you will find more. I'm also conscious of the fact that there are certain painful conditions for which, at the moment, there are no cures. The best that can be hoped for is sufficient pain reduction to give you your life back.

It's quite possible that just one therapy will solve your problem, but the philosophy behind this book is that, more often, substantial pain relief requires a combination of therapies, some making only a small contribution, but all of them together adding up to a powerful treatment. Do try them all.

I sincerely hope they'll work for you.

Paul Jenner, Spain, 2013.

What causes pain?

In this chapter you will learn:

- ▶ *that there are many different kinds of pain*
- ▶ *that the brain is at the centre of pain relief*
- ▶ *that pain can be beaten*
- ▶ *that the best way to beat pain is through a combination of techniques.*

Essentially, pain is the way your brain interprets information about a particular sensation that your body is experiencing.

Stanford School of Medicine

There are three very important things you need to know about pain.

The first is that the degree of pain you feel is in no way proportional to the seriousness of the injury or illness that you have. It's possible to feel extreme pain when there's very little, or even nothing at all, wrong. So don't go worrying that severe pain means something terrible; it probably doesn't.

The second thing you have to understand about pain is that it's not some kind of fixed system like flicking a switch in your lounge and having a light come on. It doesn't always come up with the same result. Right now you could receive a cut that rates zero on a pain scale of one to ten and yet, in a quarter of an hour, it might be a six, even though the cut is just the same.

The third thing is that the pain system itself can be attacked by germs or suffer injury, and as a result of that damage you could experience significant chronic pain, even though there's nothing otherwise wrong with your body.

So the pain system is highly fallible. You can say about pain what Winston Churchill said about democracy. It's an awful way to run things, but all the other ways are worse. In the future, technology will take over from pain, but in the meantime we have to work with the system as it is.

Oh, there's a fourth thing I should have mentioned and that's very important. Pain can be beaten. The fact that the pain system is illogical, inconsistent and fallible is very lucky for all of us. If it were perfect we'd have no chance. But its shortcomings mean it's also capable of being manipulated. That's what we'll be doing.

Imagine a burglar alarm system with various kinds of sensors – infrared motion detectors, closed circuit TV cameras, magnetic contacts on windows, pressure pads under carpets and so on. You don't want the alarm going off every time a cat passes in front of an infrared sensor. So you have a central computer that will assess the input or inputs and decide whether or not something justifies sounding the alarm.

If you were a burglar there are several things you might do to get around the alarm system. You could use a specialized infrared radiation source to 'blind' the infrared sensor. You could climb up to the alarm itself and smash it with a hammer. You could rush in and try to reprogram the central computer during the delay before the alarm went off. All kinds of things.

The pain system in the human body is very much the same and can be tackled in ways that are analogous. This book will explain how.

Assessing your pain

First of all, let's try to establish how bad your pain is and what it's actually like. It's a very difficult thing to express. Here we're going to be using a standard test known as the McGill Pain Questionnaire which does a pretty good job. It uses some rather clunky language but the meaning is fairly clear. After you've filled it in you can use your scores to help your doctor understand what you're feeling. It's also a good idea to repeat the questionnaire regularly all the time you're using the therapies in this book so you can gauge their effectiveness.

Here we go.

TABLE 1: WHAT DOES YOUR PAIN FEEL LIKE?
In each of the 20 groups of words in the table, look to see if any describe the pain you are currently experiencing. If so, circle the number of points opposite that word. Do not choose more than one word in any group; just select the single word that most applies to you. If there is no word in a group that describes your pain then do not circle any points for that group.

Group	Description	Points
1 (temporal)	flickering	1
	quivering	2
	pulsing	3
	throbbing	4
	beating	5
	pounding	6
2 (spatial)	jumping	1
	flashing	2
	shooting	3
3 (pressure)	pricking	1
	boring	2
	drilling	3
	stabbing	4
	lancing	5
4 (pressure)	sharp	1
	cutting	2
	lacerating	3
5 (pressure)	pinching	1
	pressing	2
	gnawing	3
	cramping	4
	crushing	5
6 (pressure)	tugging	1
	pulling	2
	wrenching	3
7 (thermal)	hot	1
	boring	2
	scalding	3
	searing	4
8 (brightness)	tingling	1
	itchy	2
	smarting	3
	stinging	4
9 (dullness)	dull	1
	sore	2
	hurting	3
	aching	4
	heavy	5
10 (sensory miscellaneous)	tender	1
	taut	2

	rasping	3
	splitting	4
11 (tension)	tiring	1
	exhausting	2
12 (autonomic)	sickening	1
	suffocating	2
13 (fear)	fearful	1
	frightful	2
	terrifying	3
14 (punishment)	punishing	1
	gruelling	2
	cruel	3
	vicious	4
	killing	5
15 (effective-evaluative-sensory: miscellaneous)	wretched	1
	blinding	2
16 (evaluative)	annoying	1
	troublesome	2
	miserable	3
	intense	4
	unbearable	5
17 (sensory: miscellaneous)	spreading	1
	radiating	2
	penetrating	3
	piercing	4
18 (sensory: miscellaneous)	tight	1
	numb	2
	drawing	3
	squeezing	4
	tearing	5
19 (sensory)	cool	1
	cold	2
	freezing	3
20 (affective-evaluation: miscellaneous)	nagging	1
	nauseating	2
	agonizing	3
	dreadful	4
	torturing	5

Add up all the points you've scored. The minimum is 0 and the maximum is 78.

TABLE 2: HOW STRONG IS YOUR PAIN?

Choose the most appropriate response to each question and circle the number of points opposite it. This will help your doctor understand the intensity of your pain.

Question	Response	Points
Which word describes your pain right now?	mild	1
	discomforting	2
	distressing	3
	horrible	4
	excruciating	5
Which word describes it at its worst?	mild	1
	discomforting	2
	distressing	3
	horrible	4
	excruciating	5
Which word describes it when it is least?	mild	1
	discomforting	2
	distressing	3
	horrible	4
	excruciating	5
Which word describes the worst toothache you ever had?	mild	1
	discomforting	2
	distressing	3
	horrible	4
	excruciating	5
Which word describes the worst headache you ever had?	mild	1
	discomforting	2
	distressing	3
	horrible	4
	excruciating	5
Which word describes the worst stomach ache you ever had?	mild	1
	discomforting	2
	distressing	3
	horrible	4
	excruciating	5

TABLE 3: HOW DOES YOUR PAIN CHANGE WITH TIME?

Choose the group of words that most applies to you.

Question	Response
Which word or words would you use to describe the pattern of your pain?	Continuous, steady, constant
	Rhythmic, periodic, intermittent
	Brief, momentary, transient

TABLE 4

Tell your doctor if any of the following items increase or decrease your pain

1 Alcohol

2 Stimulants such as coffee

3 Eating

4 Heat

5 Cold

6 Damp

7 Weather changes

8 Massage or use of a vibrator

9 Pressure

10 Movement

11 No movement

12 Sleep or rest

13 Lying down

14 Distraction (TV, reading etc.)

15 Urination or defecation

16 Tension

17 Bright lights

18 Loud noises

19 Going to work

20 Sexual intercourse

21 Mild exercise

22 Fatigue

Kinds of pain

So we've now got a bit of a handle on your pain, but we need to go a bit further. The more we can establish about it, the better you yourself can treat it. Your pain will fall into at least two of the following categories, which I'll be explaining in a moment:

- Acute pain

- Chronic pain

- Nociceptive pain

- Inflammatory pain

- Myofascial pain

- Neuropathic pain

- Psychogenic (psychosomatic) pain

- Breakthrough pain

- Incident pain

- Surgical pain

- Phantom pain

- Idiopathic pain

- Pathological pain

- Allodynia

- Hyperalgesia

- Dysesthesia

So let's see what those terms actually mean.

ACUTE PAIN

Acute pain is either seen as pain that stops within a specific period of time (usually six months) or as pain that goes away once the underlying problem has been cured. It's often, but not always, sharp and warns of an immediate threat to the body, either from 'external attack' by, say, heat, or from an 'internal threat' such as a disease. Nowadays we have various highly effective ways of dealing with acute pain until the body has healed itself.

CHRONIC PAIN

Chronic pain is either seen as pain that continues beyond a certain period of time (usually six months) or as pain that continues even though the underlying health problem has been cured. There is also a third way of looking at chronic pain which is that chronic pain is pain you shouldn't be feeling. Something has gone wrong with the pain system itself. Chronic pain is much more difficult to deal with than acute pain because the passing of time is no help. On the contrary, the longer chronic pain goes on the more intractable it becomes.

> ### Key idea
>
> Acute pain that's allowed to continue without treatment can easily become chronic pain that's resistant to treatment. Always tackle acute pain promptly – don't 'tough it out'.

NOCICEPTIVE PAIN

Nociceptive pain is the 'everyday' sort of pain that warns you to, say, take your fingers away from a hot saucepan. In addition to this 'superficial' pain it can also be visceral (involving the large internal organs) and deep somatic (involving the bones, ligaments, muscles and blood vessels). The process of detecting damage and relaying the information to the brain is known as nociception.

INFLAMMATORY PAIN

Inflammation is the normal response of the body to injury or disease. To you as the sufferer it seems to be part of the problem but, generally, it's part of the solution. Let's say you accidentally bang your leg really hard against a sharp object. Special cells will immediately be activated to release inflammatory mediators. These, in turn, will cause an increase in the blood supply, which is why the area reddens and feels hot to the touch. White blood cells and other components of the body's defence system will then 'leak' into the damaged tissue, thus causing the swelling. Usually the area will feel stiff. You'll be in pain because the release of a substance called bradykinin increases sensitivity. That pain has a benefit. It reminds you to protect the area from further harm until everything has been repaired. Things are slightly different if you're attacked by, say, the flu virus, because the inflammation won't be in just one place but all over your body. Your head, muscles and joints will ache. But the principle of bodily defence is the same.

So, broadly speaking, it's not a good idea to do anything to reduce inflammation. If you do, you'll be slowing down the process of recovery.

But there are also problems with inflammation. Sometimes the inflammation spreads to places it's not needed, or goes on longer than it should. Sometimes it occurs when there's no problem at all. Sometimes it compounds an existing problem, such as when inflammation caused by the flu virus destabilizes atherosclerotic plaques in coronary arteries and causes heart attacks. Sometimes it adds to an existing inflammatory condition, such as rheumatoid arthritis, elevating the pain to an intolerable level. And, sometimes, the inflammatory pain is simply too much on its own. In those situations the inflammation needs to be tackled. If you have inflammatory pain you usually won't have any problem identifying it.

Remember this

It's not the injury or the infection that causes the inflammation. The inflammation is part of the body's defence system.

MYOFASCIAL PAIN

Myofascial pain is chronic pain in the fascia or connective tissue that surrounds muscles and is due to tiny 'knots' that form when there's excessive strain, injury or, occasionally, inactivity. It's also known as myofascial pain syndrome (MPS) or chronic myofascial pain (CMP).

NEUROPATHIC PAIN

Neuropathic pain occurs when nerves send incorrect pain signals, either because the nerves have received physical damage or have become dysfunctional due to disease. In a sense it's pain you shouldn't be feeling because there's nothing wrong, except with the pain signalling system itself. It's like a burglar alarm that goes off when there's no burglar.

Peripheral neuropathy (usually affecting the hands and feet) may be due, amongst other things, to nutritional deficiencies, toxins, diabetes, cancer, HIV, herpes zoster infection and physical damage. Problems with the central nervous system may be due, amongst other things, to multiple sclerosis, strokes and physical damage to the spinal cord. In 2011, scientists from Yale University, the Veterans Affairs Medical Center, and the University of Maastricht established that mutations in the SCNA9 gene were responsible for 30 per cent of the cases of unexplained neuropathic pain.

PSYCHOGENIC (PSYCHOSOMATIC) PAIN

Psychogenic pain (also known as psychosomatic pain or psychalgia) is pain that is caused, intensified or prolonged by emotional, mental or behavioural factors. In reality, most pain includes psychogenic pain because physical pain and emotional pain activate the same areas of the brain, that's to say, the anterior insula and the anterior cingulate cortex. In practice it means that if you're already suffering emotional pain you'll feel physical pain more keenly. And if you're already in physical pain any emotional trauma will make it feel worse. Psychogenic pain is just as real, and just as terrible, as any other kind of pain but it has its own special treatment. Intriguingly, painkillers also reduce emotional pain.

BREAKTHROUGH PAIN

Breakthrough pain is the term used to describe the sensation when pain 'breaks through' medication that is being used to control it, causing sudden, short-lived distress. This especially may happen with cancer.

INCIDENT PAIN

Incident pain is the term used when pain results from movement, such as the raising of an arm.

SURGICAL PAIN

Pain following surgery may incorporate several of the previously described types of pain. In about half of cases, pain persists even after the surgical wound has completely healed.

PHANTOM PAIN

Phantom pain is pain that is felt in a part of the body that has been amputated or from which the brain no longer receives signals. It's therefore a form of neuropathic pain. Phantom pain is a terrible problem for amputees, two-thirds of whom still report it six months after the amputation. The problem is slightly worse where arms are involved as compared with lower limbs.

IDIOPATHIC PAIN

Idiopathic pain is pain that has no apparent underlying cause. That's not the same thing as saying it has no cause. The cause is not known. Fibromyalgia and irritable bowel syndrome (IBS) are often cited as idiopathic pain syndromes.

PATHOLOGICAL PAIN

Pathological pain is characterized by an amplified response either to things that normally cause no pain, or to acute pain. It therefore embraces both allodynia and hyperalgesia (below).

ALLODYNIA

Allodynia is pain due to a stimulus that does not normally provoke pain, such as a gentle caress or the pressure of clothing. Allodynia occurs when the central nervous system becomes sensitized and, at the same time, the body's own pain control mechanism (based on the release of enkephalins, endorphins and dynorphins) is no longer functioning as it should.

HYPERALGESIA

Hyperalgesia is a condition in which the sensation of pain is much stronger than it normally would be. It can be caused by nerve damage, infection, or the long-term use of opioids.

DYSESTHESIA

Dysesthesia is similar to allodynia. The sufferer may feel inappropriate pain but also any of a range of other inappropriate sensations including wetness, burning, itching, pins and needles, and something like electric shock. It's caused by lesions to the central or peripheral nervous system. Antidepressants are usually effective against dysesthesia.

Remember this

Pain is a very complicated subject and doctors and scientists don't always agree on the precise definition of the words used to describe it. You may find your doctor using some of the terms above in a slightly different way.

What exactly is pain?

So far I haven't actually said what pain is. Obviously, we all recognize it when we've got it. But although we know a great deal more about pain than we did just a generation ago we still can't precisely pin it down. Why is pain painful? We don't know. We use certain drugs very successfully against pain without even knowing how they work. So there's still quite a long way to go and several promising theories have fallen by the wayside in recent years.

What we can usefully say is that pain is your brain's interpretation of signals about things that are happening to your body. If your body was being redesigned today then, instead of pain, you might have an LED display to tell you when damage was being done. Say, an orange LED for minor damage and red for serious damage. No more pain. Sounds wonderful. But LEDs have an important defect. They're easily ignored.

Just imagine touching a very hot surface. The red LED illuminates. But you're busy concentrating on something else and it's not for three seconds that you notice the warning light. You withdraw your hand but it's already too late. Your fingertips have been incinerated.

Pain is the body's way of telling you to move your hand and it's a really good one. If you touch something hot with a fingertip you'll probably pull your hand away within about a quarter of a second. And you'll do it every time. That wouldn't happen with an LED.

In fact, it's arguable that we should feel more pain. A lot of people don't visit a dentist until they have toothache, but by then the damage may be severe. Perhaps it would be better if we felt lung pain as soon as we smoked our first cigarette, rather than after a quarter of a million when it might be too late to do anything about it.

In Stieg Larsson's Millennium Trilogy, one of the villains is a man with congenital insensitivity to pain. It makes him a formidable opponent in any fight. But in real life, such a man could not exist. Only those sufferers who take great care to avoid injury can survive. The villain got into too many fights to live very long. Infancy is a particularly dangerous time and many sufferers die very young. The fact is, if you can't feel pain you're liable to do yourself a lot of damage. Until technology comes up with something better, pain, unfortunately, is essential.

What's not essential is that you should continue to feel pain when you've taken your hand away from the heat, when the underlying problem has been cured, when you're taking action to treat the problem, when there's nothing more that can be done, or when there is no problem. That's what we'll be tackling.

Key idea

The phrase 'brain's interpretation of signals' in the explanation of pain above is a vital concept in dealing with pain. You can tackle pain by changing or suppressing those signals but you can also tackle it by modifying the interpretation.

The cumulative approach

One of your earliest experiences of pain was probably a headache. Mummy gave you some medicine and an hour later you were playing with your toys again and the pain was forgotten. Marvellous.

That's the blueprint of pain management that we all have in our minds. Take a tablet. End of problem. It's the ideal. It's what we expect our doctors to do for us.

Unfortunately, pain isn't always that simple. If it were, you wouldn't be reading this book. Quite often pain can't be tackled by a single medicament or a single anything. It needs a combined approach – lots of different things whose impact is cumulative. On their own some of those things can seem trivial. But, remember, it's not the individual effect we're interested in. It's the sum of the parts.

It's the same with so many things in life. If you were to be seeking advice on, say, climbing Mount Everest, one person might tell you to take bottled oxygen. But bottled oxygen alone isn't going to get you up Mount Everest. Another might tell you to wear a down suit. But a down suit alone isn't going to get you up Mount Everest. Yet another might recommend a long period of acclimatization at altitude. But acclimatization alone isn't going to get you up Mount Everest. It's only when these things, and many others, all come together that you can reach the summit of Mount Everest.

This book works in the same way. You may sometimes think a certain therapy seems trivial when compared with the degree of pain you're suffering. But remember, it's the combined effect of lots of things that will reduce and hopefully stop your pain. Every contribution helps. Don't disregard anything.

So let's take a brief look at these therapies. We'll be examining them in more detail as the book progresses.

NON-PRESCRIPTION AND PRESCRIPTION DRUGS

One of the first things you're going to do when pain doesn't respond to the tablets in the bathroom cupboard, or you're frightened by the pain, is see your doctor. Your doctor will listen carefully to what you have to say, consider your medical history, make a physical examination and then, almost certainly (among other things) prescribe some kind of 'painkiller' that's stronger than the one you've been using. I put painkiller in inverted commas because, nowadays, there are all kinds of medicaments, in addition to traditional analgesics, that reduce or prevent pain indirectly. So the key to medication can be to think outside the box. Look through the various kinds of drugs detailed in Chapter 2 before you go to see your doctor and discuss the options.

MIND CONTROLLED ANALGESIA

Psychological trauma damages the body physically. We all know that. We all accept, for example, that stress can lead to physical problems such as raised blood pressure. Where you may have a bit more of a problem is in accepting the idea that psychological trauma in your past can also cause physical pain *now*.

But it can.

According to one study, between 40 and 60 per cent of women and at least 20 per cent of men with chronic pain disorders report a history of being abused in childhood or adulthood. That incidence of abuse is thought to be about two to four times higher than in the general population. The abuse does not have to be sexual but if it is sexual then specific syndromes or groups of syndromes may result, including fibromyalgia and post-traumatic stress disorder.

Why should this be? According to the Alan Edwards Centre for Research on Pain at McGill University, pain experience in the first few days of life affects the way nerves develop resulting in increased pain sensitivity in later life. So that's how abuse in infancy causes problems years later. What goes on with older children and adults is less clear. What's certain (for example, in the work of J. J. Rubin) is that helping a patient to obtain an insight into the relationship between their abuse and their symptoms leads to improvement.

So there's no doubt at all that there's a link between past abuse and present pain. But we can go further. We don't have to look for anything as dramatic as abuse. Emotional pain and physical pain are closely linked. They're part of the same system. In other words, physical pain can cause emotional pain and, if it goes on long enough, it can also cause depression. In the same way, emotional pain and depression can cause physical pain or make physical pain worse.

In Chapters 3 and 4 I'll be laying out more evidence of the link between emotional pain and physical pain, explaining why the treatment of chronic pain must always include Mind Controlled Analgesia, and describing how you can successfully employ those techniques.

Key idea

The fact that some pain can be linked with emotion does not mean it's 'all in the mind'. Such pain is just as real and just as terrible as pain caused by, say, a physical injury. The significance is that (using the burglar alarm analogy) the solution will come from reprogramming the computer rather than repairing the sensors.

FOODS THAT FIGHT PAIN

According to a study for the Centers for Disease Control and Prevention in Atlanta, Georgia, foodborne diseases cause approximately 76 million illnesses in the USA every year, as well as 325,000 hospitalizations, and 5,000 deaths. But that's just the scale of the misery caused by pathogens in food. Those statistics are only scratching the surface of the problem. A far greater issue is faulty nutrition, that's to say, the food itself. Health problems related to or exacerbated by faulty nutrition include such painful conditions as heart disease, blocked arteries, kidney stones, diverticulitis, headaches and migraines, premenstrual syndrome, bad backs, rheumatoid arthritis, osteoarthritis, irritable bowel syndrome, gastroesophageal reflux disease and a third of cancers, as well as osteoporosis, high blood pressure, diabetes and impotence. That's a lot of pain and suffering. In Chapter 5 you'll learn what foods to avoid but also the foods that can actually reduce pain.

Try it now

If your pain is associated with nausea, if you have migraines, or if you have arthritis, take some fresh ginger and nibble on it. Alternatively, make an infusion with the ginger and drink it. Quite possibly you'll soon feel a little better. If you do, use ginger regularly.

SLEEP THERAPY

Yvonne C. Lee MD at Brigham and Women's Hospital in Boston led a team that compared 58 women with rheumatoid arthritis (RA) with 54 pain-free women matched by age. Using a cold water bath and an algometer (a device that can deliver a measured amount of pressure) they concluded that RA sufferers had a lower pain tolerance and pain threshold than healthy women and also an impaired ability to inhibit pain. Patients with RA had greater problems with sleep, anxiety and depression compared to controls and were more likely to exaggerate problems. Those findings are complemented by work at Israel's Rambam Medical Center (Yarnitsky D) showing that low pain inhibitory capacity is a factor in the development of idiopathic pain syndromes such as IBS and fibromyalgia. Crucially, the Boston team concluded that what's known as conditioned pain modulation (CPM) was reduced when sleep was disturbed.

In plain language it means this. If you're in pain and can't relax, and can't sleep properly, then the pain gets even worse. Eventually you can reach a point at which even light pressure can cause pain – the condition known as allodynia. It's all linked with a phenomenon called 'wind-up' in which a pain signal agitates the entire system in just the same way that one person at a football match can begin a chant which is taken up by all the supporters. As a result, pain can become magnified. So it's essential you deal with pain urgently, possibly using painkillers (Chapter 2), that you keep positive (Chapters 3 and 4) and that you teach yourself to relax and sleep (Chapter 6).

Try it now

You probably have a pretty good idea of whether you're stressed or not. However, if you're not sure try this. Place both hands on your neck. If they feel significantly colder than your neck (and assuming you haven't been playing snowballs without gloves or anything like that) you're almost certainly stressed. If they feel warm on your neck then you're relaxed.

MASSAGE THERAPY

We all instinctively rub a place that hurts, we all know the comfort of a hot water bottle, and we've all tried slapping a packet of frozen peas on a swollen ankle. But do any of these things really achieve very much in terms of pain reduction?

The answer is that they do.

Recent research has shown that massage can reduce the production of pro-inflammatory compounds known as cytokines and, at the same time, stimulate mitochondria (which provide power to your cells), helping muscles adapt to strain. Acupuncture works in a different way, stimulating the production of the body's own natural painkillers, endorphins and adenosine. As regards heat, it's been shown that it can actually deactivate pain at the molecular level in much the same way as painkilling tablets. Icing is a little more controversial because the way it reduces inflammation can inhibit healing, but it still has its place in the pain-reduction armoury. Full details are in Chapter 7.

Try it now

If you have an ache somewhere prepare a hot water bottle and hold it against the place for 10 to 15 minutes. If you don't have a hot water bottle, give the area 10 to 15 minutes of massage using a circular motion. Or try both.

EXERCISE THERAPY

Morton's toe is a common condition in which the big toe is shorter than the adjacent toe. It's that way in about 20 per cent of the population. And yet of those who seek medical help for musculoskeletal (MSK) pain, the incidence is over 80 per cent.

Why should that be?

Morton's toe causes excessive pronation, that's to say, the ankle rolls too far inwards. And that, in turn, sets off a whole chain of problems throughout the skeleton. Morton's toe demonstrates how vitally important correct posture is.

So, too, is exercise. For one thing, exercise is a way to get a shot of morphine. All you have to do is jog six miles. That's not the distance to my house or the nearest chemist. It's roughly how far you have to run for your body to generate the equivalent of a standard 10mg morphine shot. The fact is we can all produce chemicals similar to morphine. They're called endorphins (from 'endogenous' meaning 'made in the body' and 'morphine'). And exercise is one way to do it.

It may be that your medical condition doesn't permit you to exercise. But if you're capable of any exercise at all then even ten minutes is already highly beneficial in terms of endorphins. And it certainly doesn't need to be running. It could be swimming or cycling or many other fun things.

You'll find plenty of ideas on posture and exercise in Chapter 8.

Try it now

If you're able, go out and walk briskly for 10 minutes, swinging your arms and breathing deeply.

LAUGHTER THERAPY

Laughter is no laughing matter. Just as exercise does, laughter also releases endorphins, the body's own natural painkillers. In one British study led by Robin Dunbar PhD, a professor of evolutionary psychology at Oxford University, men who had been laughing at a comedy show could take up to 10 per cent more pain than other men. And it's not just a question of a direct effect on pain thresholds and tolerance. Laughter also strengthens the immune system and may therefore help cure the underlying problem. Don't worry if you're not really in a laughing mood. In Chapter 9 you'll learn that even fake laughter has a benefit.

Try it now

Find something funny on the TV or radio, or put on a humorous DVD, or download something, and have a good laugh.

ELECTRICAL AND ULTRASOUND THERAPY

Significant numbers say their pain has been reduced by Transcutaneous Electrical Nerve Stimulation (TENS) or ultrasound (or both together) and some say that it's gone completely. Most scientific studies have found these technologies to be no better than placebo but many users are convinced otherwise. Prices for the equipment for home use have fallen dramatically in recent years so these two technologies certainly come into the category 'worth a go'. They're described in Chapter 10.

MAKE A PLAN

Having read through this book you'll need to make a plan for your particular kind of pain. Keep in mind that you need to use as many different therapies as you can. Don't just opt for the one that sounds the easiest. If one thing alone works well for you then you're very lucky. It's the combined effect of several therapies together that can be so powerful. In Chapter 11 you'll find suggested programmes for particular problems.

Remember this

Even if a particular therapy only results in a 10 per cent pain reduction it's still worth including in your treatment. With half a dozen such therapies combined the total pain reduction will be substantial.

Focus points

* Severe pain does not necessarily mean that something serious is wrong – the pain system is not actually very well designed and can easily malfunction.
* Use the McGill Pain Questionnaire to help you describe your pain to your doctor and to monitor the effectiveness of the therapies you use.
* There are many different kinds of pain.
* Pain is your brain's interpretation of signals about things that are happening to your body – but we don't yet really know why pain is painful.
* Pain can be beaten.

Next step

In the next chapter we'll be looking at what will probably be your first step in combating pain, that is, the use of over the counter and prescription medicaments. If you're already on a 'painkiller' that doesn't work very well don't give up. The reality is that only some drugs – possibly only one – will be effective in your case. That's normal. The important thing is to keep trying individual drugs and combinations of drugs until you find the optimum. Everyone is different. If you prefer treatments that don't involve drugs, skip to Chapter 3.

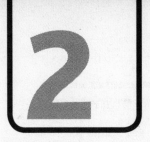

2

Non-prescription and prescription drugs

In this chapter you will learn:

▶ *how to get the best painkiller and delivery method for you*

▶ *how a drug can work for one person but not another*

▶ *why it's important to try different drugs and combinations.*

Oh! Just, subtle and mighty opium! that to the hearts of poor and rich alike, for the wounds that will never heal … bringest an assuaging balm.

Thomas De Quincey (1785–1859), English essayist.

The history of analgesic and anti-inflammatory substances goes back at least as far as the Greek and Roman physicians who used willow bark to treat fever and pain. Its use is mentioned in the Corpus Hippocraticum, a collection of medical scripts dating from around 300 BCE. As we now know, willow bark contains antioxidant, antiseptic, and antipyretic (fever reducing) compounds but especially salicin, a chemical similar to aspirin (acetylsalicylic acid).

Nowadays we have a range of painkilling drugs, the like of which Hippocrates could never even have imagined, working through a variety of different mechanisms. For sure there's a drug, or combination of drugs, that will be effective for you. The aim of this chapter is to help you find it, together with your doctor. It certainly isn't the intention of this chapter to encourage you to self-medicate. But doctors are busy people and it may take a little prompting from you to arrive at the best solution. If you try something and it doesn't work very well for you, move on to something else.

Remember this

Doctors are individuals with their own personalities. One may welcome a suggestion from you, another may resent it. You may need to employ a little 'amateur psychology' to get the best from your doctor. Never be aggressive or confrontational but do be persistent.

Key idea

The prescription of pain remedies is not yet an exact science. What works for one person may not work for another. In fact, in one study, only a third of people benefited from certain popular painkillers. You and your doctor together can only try things and see what works for you by a process of trial and error. Given that some drugs take weeks to develop their full effect, beating chronic pain can be an especially frustrating process. Have patience.

Try it now

Start a diary recording the medicament or medicaments you're taking, your degree of pain, and any symptoms and unexplained problems. Be as objective as possible. A well-kept diary will help your doctor decide what drug is best for you.

Medication overuse headaches

It's a fact that the regular use of painkillers for headaches can also cause headaches. These 'medication overuse headaches' are thought to affect about two per cent of people. Dr Mark Brown at the Department of Orthopaedics and Rehabilitation at the University of Miami explains that, 'Medications such as narcotics and or muscle relaxants cause rapid depletion of your own body's pain modulators, which makes the pain worse and prolongs the agony.' The mechanism is not well understood but it's a circular problem in which sufferers take more and more drugs to combat the headaches the drugs are causing.

According to the UK's National Institute for Health and Clinical Excellence (NICE), the level at which this happens is broadly:

▶ 15 or more days a month for aspirin, paracetamol and nonsteroidal anti-inflammatory drugs (NSAIDs)

▶ 10 or more days a month for ergots, opioids, triptans, or combination analgesics.

NICE guidelines say that if you are taking painkillers at above the threshold levels, and if they're for headaches or you're also suffering headaches along with another painful condition, then you should immediately stop for a month. However, that's a lot easier said than done. Headache is a particularly disabling kind of pain and if you could manage without painkillers you probably would have done so.

As an alternative to painkillers, NICE recommends acupuncture for chronic tension-type headaches and migraine. If that doesn't work, the European Federation of Neurological Societies (EFNS) says topiramate, an anticonvulsant (see Prescription Drugs below) is the only medicament that's effective for both migraine and medication overuse. As regards withdrawal symptoms, the EFNS rates the corticosteroids prednisone, prednisolone and amitriptyline as 'possibly effective'.

Case study

'I've been getting two or three migraines a week for the past few years. I'm on various medications. Recently the number of attacks has been creeping up and I've been getting more and more side effects. So I decided to stop taking all medications to see what would happen. I found I could sometimes tough it out by doing things like taking a shower and leaving my hair wet, which seems to help. Over a couple of months I concluded that two of the medications were definitely helping and the rest weren't. Working with my doctor I switched to a substitute for one of the effective drugs and I'm now having fewer side effects. You have to keep trying different things to see what works for you and what doesn't.' Melanie (27)

Key idea

The World Health Organization recommends that analgesics should be taken 'by the clock', that's to say, at regular intervals (usually every three to six hours), rather than 'on demand' (meaning when the pain becomes too much).

Delivery methods

Numerous delivery methods are possible:

▶ Pills and capsules. This is the method everyone is familiar with. The disadvantage is that drugs administered via the digestive tract are slow to act and, if your condition makes you vomit, some or all of the medicine may be lost.

▶ Sublingual tablets. Held under the tongue, these tablets act faster than tablets that are swallowed.

▶ Nasal sprays. Nasal sprays are even faster than sublingual tablets but it can take practice to do it right. In the UK, the non-prescription sumatriptan, for migraines, comes as a spray.

▶ Suppositories. Suppositories work about as fast as nasal sprays, the drug being absorbed through the rectal lining.

▶ Injections. Injection can place a drug precisely where it's needed. For osteoarthritis, for example, hyaluronic acid or corticosteroid may be injected directly into a joint, while for muscle pain, a local anaesthetic and/or a corticosteroid may be injected into a trigger point.

▶ Self-injection. For severe, rapid headaches self-injection is the fastest method of gaining relief.

▶ Skin patches. The advantage of skin patches, when used for the delivery of opioid painkillers, is that they provide continuous relief from chronic, severe pain (caused by cancer, for example) and last for 72 to 96 hours, depending on the type.

▶ Creams. For joint and muscle pain, topical analgesic creams have the advantage that they can be applied directly to the area that hurts. Since the chemicals don't have to pass through the stomach, gastrointestinal side effects are reduced. Ultrasound can speed absorption (see Chapter 10).

Key idea

The same drug can have different effects depending on the delivery method used, so discuss the options with your doctor. Side effects may also vary.

The following information is given to alert you to the many drug options that now exist. Because drugs can be sold under a huge variety of brand names, depending on the manufacturer and the country, the descriptions that follow use the chemical names of the drugs, which are the same everywhere. The information about doses is given as a guide to the sort of regime you'll need to follow if you opt for a particular drug. In the case of non-prescription drugs you should read the accompanying information leaflet very carefully and follow the dosing advice given there. If your doctor prescribes a drug then you should take the dose he or she stipulates. There isn't space in a book of this size to list every possible side effect of the drugs described and only the most common, significant side effects are given. For full details consult the information leaflet provided with the medicament. If you have concerns, discuss them with your doctor.

Remember this

It's dangerous to exceed the maximum recommended dose.

Non-prescription drugs

Regulations vary from country to country. The following are painkillers that are generally available without prescription but, in certain countries, a prescription may nevertheless be required.

ACETAMINOPHEN – SEE PARACETAMOL

ASPIRIN

▶ **What will it do for me?**

Aspirin (acetylsalicylic acid) is an analgesic, an anti-inflammatory and an antipyretic (reduces fever). It's effective against minor aches and pains. At low doses it also lowers the risk of blood clots, strokes and heart attacks and may help prevent colorectal cancer. Aspirin belongs to the nonsteroidal anti-inflammatory (NSAID) group of painkillers (see below). Salicylic acid, into which aspirin is converted in the body, is contained in many fruits and some vegetables and can also be made in the body.

▶ **How should I use it?**

The standard dose is around 300 mg four times a day. For the prevention of heart disease the recommended dose is around 80 mg once a day.

▶ **Any side effects?**

Aspirin has a high risk of stomach ulcers. Some people have an intolerance to salicylic acid which can manifest in various ways including skin rashes, angioedema (swelling in the deep layers of the skin), asthma, frequent urination and headaches. If you are intolerant of aspirin you should also avoid other NSAIDs. It should not be given to children due to the risk of Reye's syndrome, which can be fatal.

CODEINE

▶ What will it do for me?

Codeine (3-methylmorphine) is at the weak end of the opioid range and is suitable for mild to moderate pain. In a study of 38 oral analgesics for surgical pain, led by Andrew Moore at the Oxford Pain Research Unit, codeine was the least effective. It is also sometimes used to treat diarrhoea. In the UK codeine is only available without prescription as a weak ingredient together with another painkiller such as paracetamol. In the USA, regulations vary from state to state but, in general, if codeine is available at all without prescription then it is as a weak ingredient along with other painkillers. In other countries laws vary enormously.

▶ How should I use it?

The standard adult dose for pain relief is 30 mg every six hours; doses up to 60 mg every four hours have been used.

▶ Any side effects?

The most common side effects include drowsiness and constipation. Serious side effects from occasional use are rare. A small percentage of people have allergic reactions causing skin rashes and swellings. Do not take codeine together with alcohol.

MENTHOL

▶ What will it do for me?

Rubbed into the skin, menthol increases blood circulation, creates a soothing sensation and also has local analgesic properties, making it useful for muscle and joint pain, nerve pain, and headaches.

▶ How should I use it?

Menthol is available in the form of lotions, gels, creams and deodorant-type sticks and roll-ons. It can be used freely.

Any side effects?

Some menthol preparations also include an analgesic so check the label carefully for anything to which you might be allergic. Test the product on a tiny area of skin first. Don't use on broken skin or get menthol in your eyes.

NEURAGEN PN®

▶ What will it do for me?

Unlike the other chemicals described in this chapter, Neuragen PN is a branded product but, because effective treatments for neuropathic pain are so few, I've decided to include it. How effective is it? In one randomized, double blind, placebo controlled clinical trial of patients with neuropathic pain, over 90 per cent reported pain reduction within 30 minutes of applying it. There is some suggestion that the pleasant scent may have influenced the results but it seems to be something worth trying. Neuragen PN combines St John's Wort, Wolfsbane, Club Moss, Poison Ivy and Rye ergot in a blend of five plant oils. Which ingredients are effective is unknown but one of the five oils, geranium oil, has been shown to have some effect on neuropathic pain on its own.

▶ How should I use it?

Neuragen PN can be applied to the skin as required.

▶ Any side effects?

Geranium oil can cause rashes, a burning sensation, eye irritation and light headedness while long-term use of the oils may have other harmful effects. As a precaution, Neuragen PN should not be used by children, or women who are pregnant or breastfeeding.

NONSTEROIDAL ANTI-INFLAMMATORY DRUGS (NSAIDs)

▶ What will they do for me?

NSAIDs are effective painkillers generally and especially useful when the pain is associated with inflammation (as with some types of back ache) because of their anti-inflammatory effects. The common oral NSAIDs are ibuprofen, naproxen, and aspirin (which has been given its own entry). Naproxen is prescription-only in many countries but may be bought over the counter (OTC) in the USA and the UK (where it is sold under the brand name Feminax Ultra® as it's particularly useful for dysmenorrhea or painful periods). The NSAID diclofenac is often used as a gel for local use on arthritic joints.

▶ How should I use it?

In the case of ibuprofen, take 400 mg – 600 mg every six hours, preferably with meals, with a maximum of 1,600 mg a day. In the case of naproxen, the standard dose is 250 mg – 500 mg (or 275 mg – 550 mg of naproxen sodium) twice a day, but in certain cases the dose may be higher. Don't exceed 1,500 mg of naproxen in 24 hours. If you need to take NSAIDs for a prolonged period take one day off each week – you should still have enough circulating in your body to keep the pain at bay.

▶ Any side effects?

NSAIDs block prostaglandin PGE_2 and certain other substances that, as one of their many functions, protect the stomach by stimulating mucus production and inhibiting the secretion of stomach acid. They thus open the door to pain and ulcers and may exacerbate inflammatory bowel disease. The risk increases with the use of alcohol and tobacco. Taking a proton pump inhibitor (such as omeprazole) to suppress acid production offers some protection. Prolonged use can cause kidney problems, especially in those with diabetes. A study published in the British Medical Journal in January 2011, covering 116,000 patients, concluded that regular, long-term use of NSAIDs at high doses increased the risk of heart attacks and tripled the risk of strokes (note that naproxen carries a 50 per cent lower risk than ibuprofen). Regular use of NSAIDs for three months or more increases the risk of erectile dysfunction by a factor of 1.4, according to one study. Do not take NSAIDs if you are pregnant or allergic to aspirin.

Key idea

In addition to other side effects, painkillers can sometimes cause allergic reactions. They may include skin rashes and swelling and, in extreme cases, anaphylactic shock which, if not promptly treated, can be fatal.

If you have significant swelling of the tongue after taking a medication get medical help immediately. In the general population about one per cent of people are thought to be allergic to non-steroidal anti-inflammatory drugs (NSAIDs), but if you have asthma your likelihood of allergy to NSAIDs will be higher.

PARACETAMOL (ACETAMINOPHEN)

▶ What will it do for me?

Paracetamol (or acetaminophen in the USA) works by raising the pain threshold. In other words, if there's only mild pain you'll no longer feel it. Relief begins after about half an hour and lasts for three to four hours.

▶ How should I use it?

Adults can take up to 1,000 mg three times a day, preferably half an hour before a meal or two hours after. If you're also taking a cold or flu remedy check to see if it contains paracetamol – if so, make sure the combined dose is within the recommended limit. If you need to continue for more than a week don't exceed 2,000 mg a day.

▶ Any side effects?

Paracetamol is generally safe at the recommended dose, but overdoses could cause serious and even fatal liver damage. In rare cases severe liver damage has occurred at the normal dose. Alcoholism increases the risk. Other possible side effects are stomach pains, fatigue and light-headedness.

TRIPTAN

▶ What will it do for me?

Triptans are the drug of choice for many migraine sufferers, stopping attacks or at least reducing the symptoms, within 30 to 90 minutes in 70 to 80 per cent of people. They're also used for cluster headaches. Triptans are a family of tryptamine-based drugs that act on serotonin receptors in nerve endings and blood vessels. They're generally only available on prescription but in the UK sumatriptan was made an over-the-counter (OTC) drug in 2006 under the brand name Imigran Recovery®.

▶ How should I use it?

The standard dose is a single 50 mg sumatriptan tablet taken as soon as possible after the start of an attack.

▶ Any side effects?

Common side effects are tingling, drowsiness, dizziness, flushing (from a short-term increase in blood pressure), nausea, and fatigue. Triptans aren't recommended for those at risk of heart attacks or strokes. Triptans should not be taken by those on selective serotonin reuptake inhibitors (SSRIs) or selective serotonin/norepinephrine reuptake inhibitors (SNRIs) without medical advice.

Key idea

If you develop a medical problem in the days or weeks after starting a new medication it's all too easy to attribute it to the new drug. It's also the case that when you look for side effects you're likely to find them. Try not to jump to conclusions.

Try it now

You're not the only one wrestling with the choice of medicaments, their effectiveness and side effects. Put the name of your drug into your internet search engine together with the word 'forum' to see what experiences other people are having.

Prescription drugs

A huge range of prescription drugs is available nowadays for the treatment of pain. That means you'll only be able to have one or more of those drugs if your doctor agrees. Take a little time to read through the descriptions below and identify the drugs you think may work best for you. Note that some are painkillers while others (such as beta-blockers for migraine) have no painkilling ability whatsoever but can prevent the events that cause the pain. Make a list of possible drugs and then discuss them with your doctor.

Tell your doctor clearly how much pain you're in. Use the McGill Pain Questionnaire in Chapter 1 to help you. Try not to be too emotional, or you run the risk that some aspect of your pain will be put down to 'neurosis'.

Don't be aggressive but do be assertive. Use the following three-part structure to acknowledge your doctor's point of view (about side effects, for example), to state your own position and, finally, to make a proposal that takes account of both. For example, if you would like more powerful painkillers you might say something like this:

1 I fully understand your reservations about the addictive nature of opioids.

2 However, I'm in such pain that I can't enjoy anything or even carry out basic tasks.

3 Couldn't I at least try an opioid to see what difference it makes to my quality of life?

Your doctor will probably be working to the 'analgesic ladder' which basically means progressing from the weakest painkillers with the fewest side effects towards the strongest with the most significant side effects. Here's the ladder:

▶ Simple analgesics (such as paracetamol and NSAIDs)

▶ Weak opioids (such as codeine)

▶ Strong opioids (such as morphine)

▶ Indirect painkillers (drugs not originally intended for pain, such as anticonvulsants).

Obviously it makes sense to avoid the possibility of harmful side effects and you may have to be patient if you think you need very strong drugs.

Remember this

Do not self-medicate with prescription drugs bought on the internet. They're prescription-only for a good reason. It requires the expertise of a trained medical practitioner to judge what's suitable for you given your age, state of health, gender, possible drug interactions and so on. It's also the case that many medicines sold over the internet are bogus. Be safe by consulting your doctor and following his or her advice.

Key idea

Most prescription drugs have an alarming list of possible side effects. But that doesn't mean you'll experience any of them. It's simply a fact of life that some people will be susceptible and the pharmaceutical companies have to take account of that. If you have concerns, discuss them with your doctor.

ANTICONVULSANTS (NERVE MEMBRANE STABILIZERS)

▶ What will they do for me?

Anticonvulsants, such as gabapentin (also known as nerve membrane stabilizers) were originally designed to treat epilepsy but they also relieve nerve pain. They work by boosting the neurotransmitter GABA (gamma-aminobutyric acid), a deficiency of which causes increased pain, anxiety, irritability, headaches – and seizures. There are a number of different compounds in this class of drugs and if one doesn't work well for you another may do better. Gabapentin, for example, is effective for allodynia (pain in response to a stimulus that does not normally cause pain), hyperesthesia (increased sensitivity to pain), burning pain and shooting pains. Pregabalin works well for fibromyalgia.

▶ How should I use it?

For gabapentin you'll need to build up to the maintenance dose by taking 300 mg on the first day, 300 mg twice a day on the second day, and 300 mg three times a day on the third day. Thereafter the maintenance dose is from 300 mg to 600 mg three times a day (900 mg to 1800 mg in total a day). In the case of pregabalin, the standard dose is one capsule two or three times a day.

▶ Any side effects?

As regards gabapentin, studies conducted to date have found that it's generally tolerated very well, but if you have kidney problems the dose may need to be reduced. As regards pregabalin, the list of possible side effects is long and includes skin problems, chest or muscle pain, blurred vision, swelling of the extremities and lack of coordination. Most seriously, it can cause mental health problems.

ANTIDEPRESSANTS

▶ What will they do for me?

Tricyclic antidepressants such as amitriptyline have been found to be effective for nerve pain (as with shingles and sciatica, for example). The fact that you are prescribed amitriptyline does not mean the doctor believes your pain is psychological – its method of acting on pain is something quite separate. One in three sufferers of chronic pain will get better than 50 per cent relief. Note that the benefit does not begin immediately and it could take up to two weeks before you notice any difference and possibly as long as two months to get the full effect.

▶ How should I use it?

With amitriptyline your doctor will probably start you on 10 mg to 25 mg a day, from where you'll gradually build up, if necessary, to 100 mg a day.

▶ Any side effects?

Dizziness and sleepiness. If that is the case with you, take the tablet (or syrup) a couple of hours before going to bed. Amitriptyline doesn't work for everyone but some people are very happy with it and use it for years.

BETA-BLOCKERS

▶ What will they do for me?

Beta-blockers such as propranolol are primarily prescribed for angina, high blood pressure, irregular heartbeat and heart attack. But, taken daily, they also prevent or reduce the frequency of migraine attacks, cluster headaches and tension headaches in some people.

▶ How should I use it?

The standard dose for propranolol is usually 80 mg a day but in some circumstances up to 240 mg a day might be prescribed. Because of the possible side effects it's normal to begin on a lower dose (10 mg to 30 mg) and work up. The full benefit of propranolol in the treatment of headaches may take as much as three months to develop.

▶ Any side effects?

Common side effects of propranolol include insomnia, fatigue, dizziness, upset stomach, flatulence, cramping, vomiting, rashes, cold hands and feet, reduced sex drive, diarrhoea and constipation. It usually takes two to four weeks for the body to adjust and for the side effects to go away. Propranolol can reduce blood sugar and may therefore be unsuitable for diabetics. It is not recommended during pregnancy or if breastfeeding. It interacts with an extensive range of other drugs, so make sure your doctor is aware of every medicament that you're taking. Propranolol should never be stopped abruptly as chest pains may result.

BIOLOGIC RESPONSE MODIFIERS

▶ What will they do for me?

Often used together with DMARDs (see below) for the treatment of rheumatoid arthritis, biologic response modifiers, such as etanercept, target various protein molecules to inhibit the immune response. They had also been seen as a safe treatment for back pain but a study of 84 sufferers published in the 'Annals of Internal Medicine' in 2012 concluded that the biologic etanercept was less effective than steroids after one month and about as effective as placebo after six months.

▶ How should I use it?

Etanercept is injected subcutaneously, usually once a week.

▶ Any side effects?

All of this group of drugs are powerful immunosuppressants and some patients have experienced serious and sometimes fatal side effects.

BOTULINUM TOXIN

▶ What will it do for me?

Injected into the muscles of the head and neck, Botulinum toxin type A (Botox) was approved by the American FDA as a treatment for chronic migraines in 2010. It seems to be effective for some people but others derive no benefit.

► How should I use it?

Botulinum toxin is produced by the *Clostridium botulinum* bacteria and is the most toxic substance known. Because of the potential danger and the need for absolute precision it should only be administered by a properly qualified and experienced person. The injections need to be repeated every 12 weeks.

► Any side effects?

Most seriously, there have been deaths attributed to the use of Botox as a result of it spreading to other areas of the body. However, in terms of the percentage of deaths relative to the use of Botox both medically and cosmetically the risk is tiny. More common side effects include bruising and swelling at the site of the injections, allergy, difficulty swallowing, flu-like symptoms and fatigue.

Remember this

Following Botox injections, avoid rubbing or massaging the area because of the risk of the toxin spreading.

BUTALBITAL

► What will it do for me?

Butalbital is a barbiturate, that's to say, a drug that acts as a central nervous system depressant. For the treatment of pain, especially headaches, it's normally combined with other medicaments. Fioricet®, for example, is a combination of butalbital, paracetamol (acetaminophen) and caffeine. Other combinations include aspirin and codeine. Many migraine sufferers find butalbital combinations particularly effective.

► How should I use it?

The standard dose for Fioricet is one or two tablets every four hours with a maximum of six tablets in 24 hours.

► Any side effects?

The most common side effects of butalbital include drowsiness, dizziness, nausea, abdominal pain, and feeling lightheaded. Above all, butalbital is addictive and although butalbital combinations are available in the USA they're not in the UK.

CALCIUM CHANNEL BLOCKERS

► What will they do for me?

Calcium channel blockers do exactly what they say. They prevent calcium from entering the blood vessel walls and heart, thereby reducing blood pressure. They're effective for some kinds of migraine and for angina (chest pain).

► How should I use it?

Some calcium channel blockers last only a few hours while others are designed to release slowly. Doses vary depending on the actual medication. For the prevention of migraine attacks, the standard dose of verapamil is 80 mg three to four times a day.

► Any side effects?

Side effects are generally minor, including dizziness, drowsiness, nausea, headache, constipation, rapid heartbeat and swelling of the feet and ankles. Do not take calcium channel blockers with grapefruit or grapefruit products.

CANNABIS

► What will it do for me?

Cannabis has been in use for, perhaps, five thousand years. A study by Oxford University's Centre for Functional Magnetic Resonance Imaging of the Brain found that THC (the most studied of the 400 active ingredients in cannabis) didn't actually reduce pain but could alter the emotional response to it. Some people felt detached from the pain and were less bothered by it (thus chemically achieving the same result as Acceptance and Commitment Therapy – see Chapter 4). Researchers like Dr Willy Notcutt at James Paget hospital, Great Yarmouth, have found it particularly useful for patients suffering from multiple sclerosis.

Because of its use as a recreational drug, cannabis is tightly controlled or even banned in many countries. In the UK, Sativex®, which is sprayed into the mouth, became the first cannabis-based prescription medicine in the world in 2010. In Canada, marijuana is permitted medicinally for those with debilitating and grave illnesses. In the USA at the time of writing, some 20 states allow cannabis for medical purposes and two states, Washington and Colorado, have legalized it for recreational use in certain circumstances. But these states are in conflict with federal law.

▶ How should I use it?

Sativex users should begin with one spray in the evening on the first day and, if necessary, work up to the maximum of 12 sprays over a two week period. If you live somewhere that cannabis is legal and you smoke it then the dose is up to you, but take note of the side effects.

▶ Any side effects?

The most common side effects of Sativex are dizziness and fatigue. Care should be taken when combining it with other medicaments that cause sleepiness. Cannabis in any form should not be used by women who are pregnant or breastfeeding, or by those with psychiatric disorders (other than depression). Youngsters smoking cannabis run an increased risk of developing a psychotic illness, and in the case of skunk (an especially potent variety) the risk is substantial. Smoking cannabis together with tobacco introduces the chance of, among other things, heart disease and cancer.

Remember this

If your doctor doesn't seem to be very experienced in pain management, ask to be referred to a specialist pain clinic. These exist in the USA, the UK and many other countries.

CORTICOSTEROIDS

▶ What will they do for me?

Not to be confused with the bodybuilder's anabolic steroids, corticosteroids are powerful anti-inflammatory drugs. They may be used for the treatment of arthritis, as well as asthma, autoimmune diseases such as multiple sclerosis, certain skin conditions such as eczema, and some kinds of cancer. The corticosteroid dexamethasone is sometimes used together with other migraine drugs to improve pain relief.

▶ How should I use it?

Because of the side effects, oral corticosteroids (also known as oral catabolic steroids) should ideally only be used for short periods, with a maximum of two weeks. Your doctor will probably start you off on a high dose to relieve the pain and then move to a lower dose for a few days. Corticosteroids may also be injected directly into a painful joint, giving relief that may last from weeks to months.

▶ Any side effects?

In the long term, oral corticosteroids can cause osteoporosis, collapse of the hip joint, weight gain, stomach ulcers and cataracts. A single injection is unlikely to have significant side effects but frequent injections may cause joint damage.

DISEASE-MODIFYING ANTIRHEUMATIC DRUGS (DMARDs)

▶ What will they do for me?

Disease-modifying antirheumatic drugs (DMARDs) prevent or slow the attack on joints in rheumatoid arthritis. They're often used in conjunction with biologic response modifiers (see above). Via a different mechanism, DMARDs are also used as chemotherapy drugs to fight cancer.

▶ How should I use it?

Oral doses are taken weekly. Low doses are used for rheumatoid arthritis, high doses for chemotherapy.

▶ Any side effects?

In low doses for rheumatoid arthritis DMARDs are fairly safe but side effects may still include hair loss, headaches, nausea and skin pigmentation problems. In high chemotherapy doses additional side effects include abdominal pain, dizziness, fatigue, fever and low white blood cell count (thus increasing the risk of infections).

ERGOTS

▶ What will they do for me?

In the past, drugs combining ergotamine and caffeine (such as Cafergot® and Migergot®) have been prescribed to stop migraine attacks. They work by arresting the dilation of blood vessels and therefore need to be taken immediately at the onset of symptoms. If taken later they have no effect. Certain individuals prefer them to all other migraine drugs but, in general, they're less effective than triptans. Recently concerns about the safety of ergots has led to them becoming unavailable in many countries.

▶ How should I use it?

Cafergot, where available, comes in tablets of 1mg ergotamine tartrate/100 mg caffeine. The dose is two tablets at the first sign of an attack, with one additional tablet every half hour if necessary, up to a maximum of six tablets per attack or 10 tablets a week.

▶ Any side effects?

There is a high risk of ergot poisoning for which the early signs include nausea, vomiting, muscle pain, weakness, numbness, itching, and either slow or rapid heartbeat. Symptoms may then progress to vision problems, dizziness, confusion, convulsions and, finally, death. If you suspect ergot poisoning seek immediate medical attention.

FLUPIRTINE

▶ What will it do for me?

Flupirtine is unique in being a non-NSAID, non-steroidal, non-opioid analgesic. It suppresses pain perception transmission in the brain and spinal cord and works best for non-inflammatory conditions. Nevertheless, because of its muscle relaxant properties it is popular for back pain. It's also used for migraines, cancer pain, postoperative pain and gynaecological problems and has shown promise against fibromyalgia. It also appears to have neuro-protective properties in the case of Creutzfeld-Jakob disease, Alzheimer's disease and multiple sclerosis. Flupirtine first became available in Europe in 1984 but, at the time of writing, is not available in either the USA or the UK.

▶ How should I use it?

The standard oral dose is 100 mg three or four times a day. It can also be taken as a suppository.

▶ Any side effects?

The most common side effects are dizziness, drowsiness, dry mouth and nausea. Less commonly there may be liver toxicity and cardiac issues. Flupirtine is non-addictive and there seems to be little or no build-up of tolerance.

HYALURONIC ACID

▶ What will it do for me?

Injected into painful joints, hyaluronic acid boosts the natural shock absorbency. Studies have found it to be about as effective as NSAIDs for some people with osteoarthritis, with relief lasting from six months to a year. But it's not effective for everyone.

▶ How should I use it?

Depending on the brand, you may receive just one injection or three to five at weekly intervals.

▶ Any side effects?

Don't do any serious weight-bearing exercise for a couple of days.

LOCAL ANAESTHETICS

▶ What will they do for me?

Local anaesthetics, given by injection, drip or cream, can substantially or completely numb the pain from a specific area. They're mostly used for surgical procedures but also by professional athletes to allow an early return to play. The only form that's widely available is the lidocaine patch which is applied to the skin. It was originally designed to treat postherpetic neuralgia (PHN), that's to say, the pain caused by shingles, but has also proven useful for low-back pain. In one study, 29 per cent of PHN sufferers reported 'a lot' or 'complete' relief while 53 per cent reported 'moderate or better' pain relief.

▶ How should I use it?

The standard patch is 5 per cent lidocaine and can be worn for up to 12 hours in any 24 hour period. In other words, there must be a 12 hour break between patches.

▶ Any side effects?

Lidocaine patches may cause drowsiness, dizziness or blurred vision. Seek medical advice if you're pregnant, trying to become pregnant, breastfeeding, have liver or kidney problems, or taking other medicines, especially beta-blockers or antiarrhythmics.

MUSCLE RELAXANTS

▶ What will they do for me?

Muscle relaxants are often prescribed at the beginning of a course of back pain treatment as a short-term measure. There are several different kinds but they all act on the brain rather than directly on the muscles to prevent muscle spasms.

▶ How should I use it?

The standard dose for carisoprodol is 350 mg every eight hours, for cyclobenzaprine 10 mg every six hours, and for diazepam (better known as Valium®) 5–10 mg every six hours.

▶ Any side effects?

Carisoprodol can cause dependence; cyclobenzaprine can cause confusion and, in men with enlarged prostates, urinary retention; diazepam is a depressant and can worsen the depression that may be associated with chronic pain – it also disturbs sleep patterns leading to insomnia once the course of treatment is over.

NONSTEROIDAL ANTI-INFLAMMATORY DRUGS (NSAIDs)

▶ What will they do for me?

Non-prescription NSAIDs have already been described above. Prescription versions generally have stronger painkilling abilities but also a greater risk of side effects. One, however, is worth mentioning specifically and that's celecoxib (brand name Celebrex®) because it blocks the enzyme cyclooxygenase-2

(COX-2) that causes inflammation, but unlike other NSAIDs, doesn't block cyclooxygenase-1 (COX-1) that protects the stomach. Celecoxib is therefore safer in terms of gastrointestinal damage but there's controversy over the risk of cardiovascular problems. In a study of 38 oral analgesics for surgical pain led by Andrew Moore at the Oxford Pain Research Unit, the NSAID etoricoxib came out on top but is considered to have significant risks and is not available everywhere.

▶ How should I use it?

There are too many prescription NSAIDs to give the dosages here. Follow your doctor's advice.

▶ Any side effects?

Although all NSAIDs have broadly the same kinds of risks, the degree of risk for any given side effect varies from one to another. In one study, rofecoxib and celecoxib, for example, had an increased risk of death of 1.7, while for diclofenac the increase in risk was of the order of 2.1. As regards gastrointestinal side effects, celecoxib, nabumetone, ibuprofen and diclofenac have the lowest rates, while indomethacin, ketoprofen and piroxicam have a high prevalence.

OPIOID DRUGS

▶ What will they do for me?

Derived from the opium poppy, the opioid group contains the most powerful known painkillers, the most potent of which is more than a million times stronger than aspirin. The most famous of the group is morphine which has a duration of around three to four hours when given by the intravenous, intramuscular or subcutaneous routes, and around three to six hours when given by mouth. Opioid painkillers can also be absorbed transdermally through the use of skin patches, the effect lasting for up to three days.

▶ How should I use it?

That depends on the opioid – see the table below for relative strengths. Some opioid painkillers are a mixture with paracetamol (acetaminophen). If so, the acetaminophen should be limited to 3,000 mg per day.

▶ Any side effects?

The problem with opioids is that they're highly likely to cause dependence and that's why your doctor will be reluctant to prescribe them. In the USA, the use of oxycodone and hydrocodone is said to have reached epidemic proportions. It's believed that approaching two million Americans are either abusing painkillers or are dependent on them or addicted to them. And according to the US Department of Health and Human Services, over six million Americans are using prescription drugs for non-medical reasons.

Common side effects of opioids include drowsiness, dizziness, headache, nausea, vomiting, constipation, diarrhoea, anxiety, tremors and a reduction in beneficial REM sleep. Other possible side effects include hallucinations and, paradoxically, hyperalgesia (increased sensitivity to pain) which, in rare cases, has begun after as little as one month's use. Long-term use can interfere with sex hormones leading to loss of libido, infertility and an increased risk of osteoporosis.

Nevertheless, in many ways, opioids are safer than other kinds of painkillers.

▶ Opioids and their relative strengths

Analgesic/opioid	Strength relative to morphine	Dose equivalent to 10 mg morphine
Morphine (oral)	1	10 mg
Aspirin (non-opioid)	1/360	No equivalent dose
Diflunisal (NSAID, non opioid)	1/160	1600 mg
Paracetamol/Acetaminophen	1/25	250 mg
Codeine	1/10	100 mg
Tramadol	1/10	100mg
Anileridine	1/4	40 mg
Pethidine	0.36	28 mg
Hydrocodone	0.60	17 mg
Oxycodone	1.5 – 2.0	5.0 – 6.7 mg
Methadone (acute)	3.0 – 4.0	2.5 – 3.3 mg
Morphine (IV/IM*)	4.0	2.5 mg
Diamorphine (Heroin; IV/IM)	1.9 – 4.3	2.3 – 5.2 mg
Hydromorphone	5.0	2.0 mg
Oxymorphone	7.0	1.4 mg

Methadone (chronic)	7.5	1.35 mg
Levorphanol	8.0	1.3 mg
Buprenorphine	40.0	0.25 mg
Fentanyl	50 – 100	0.1 – 0.2 mg
Sufentanil	500 – 1,000	10 – 20 μg
Etorphine	1,000 – 3,000	3.3 – 10 μg
Carfentanil	10,000 – 100,000	0.1 – 1.0 μg

Notes: IV = intravenous; IM = intramuscular.

▶ How can I come off opioid painkillers?

Coming off opioids after medium to long-term use can be difficult. That doesn't mean you're addicted in the true sense of the word. The true addict is someone who wants to continue taking the substance even though there's no medical reason. You do want to stop and, of course, you will. But don't go 'cold turkey' – that's to say, don't stop abruptly. Your body needs time to adjust and it will be better to taper off the dose. This is something you need to discuss with your doctor because procedures vary according to your situation, the opioid you have been taking, and for how long.

Let's say you had surgery on your back and have been taking two hydrocodone/paracetamol tablets every six hours, making eight tablets a day.

▶ Slow taper: reduce by one tablet every three days (in which case you would be off the medication in three weeks).

▶ Fast taper: reduce to one tablet every six hours on the first day, one tablet every eight hours for three days, one tablet every 12 hours for three days and one tablet every 24 hours for three days (in which case you would be off the medication in 10 days).

Withdrawal symptoms from cutting down too quickly might be some of the following:

▶ Abdominal cramps

▶ Anxiety

▶ Diarrhoea

▶ Dilated pupils

- Goose bumps
- Hypertension
- Insomnia
- Muscle twitching
- Runny nose
- Rapid heartbeat
- Rapid breathing
- Sweating
- Weakness

Do opioids hasten death?

There's a general belief, also held by some members of the medical profession, that the use of morphine and other opioids, hastens death in the elderly and terminally ill. But various studies (for example, Thorns A., Sykes N.) have not found that to be the case.

Remember this

When you're in pain it's very tempting to ask for the strongest analgesic that exists. You want the pain to end and you want it to end immediately. But as a general rule, the stronger the painkiller the more serious the side effects. It makes sense to begin with the least dangerous and combine it with the other kinds of therapies described in this book.

TRIPTAN

What will it do for me?

Triptans, the drug of choice for many migraine sufferers, were dealt with under non-prescription painkillers above.

Key idea

Quite possibly your doctor will prescribe two or even three drugs. This is known as multi-modal analgesia. The idea is to maximize pain relief while minimizing side effects

Try it now

If you're having a problem with your medication, because it's ineffective or because it has too many side effects, make an appointment with your doctor right now to review the situation. Before you go, read through this chapter once more, making a note of the classes of drugs that might be helpful in your case.

Focus points

✱ A huge variety of drugs is now available for the relief of pain – if something doesn't work for you, ask your doctor to try a different drug or combination.

✱ It's possible for painkillers to become the cause of pain, a phenomenon known as 'medication overuse headache'.

✱ Opioids include the most powerful known painkillers, but they carry a high risk of dependence and addiction.

✱ Don't self-medicate with drugs bought on the internet.

✱ Don't rely on drugs alone for the prevention of or relief of pain – use them as necessary in combination with the other methods described in this book.

Next step

Drugs are the quickest and most certain way of gaining relief from pain but, as we've seen in this chapter, they all have side effects and some of those side effects are serious. In the rest of this book we'll be looking at ways of beating pain that have no side effects and that may, in certain cases, cure the underlying problem. The first of these techniques, described in the next chapter, are Neuro-Linguistic Programming (NLP) and self-hypnosis.

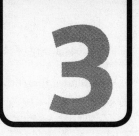

Mind Controlled Analgesia

In this chapter you will learn:

▶ *the techniques of Mind Controlled Analgesia (MCA)*

▶ *how to reduce pain through visualization*

▶ *how to hypnotize yourself.*

Pain has a way of clipping our wings and keeping us from being able to fly … and if left unresolved for very long, you can almost forget that you were ever created to fly in the first place.

Wm. Paul Young, The Shack

Here's an interesting little experiment. At this moment, can you hear the blood circulating through your left ear? I'm assuming that you can't. Now focus all your attention on that ear. It will help to close your eyes and swivel them to the left. Spend two or three minutes concentrating on this task.

So how did you get on? Almost certainly you could hear the blood pulsing. And that tells you something very interesting about the mind-body connection and pain. You have the capability to increase your sensitivity to your body and, by the same token, you have the ability to decrease it. In other words, to increase and decrease the sensation of pain.

Now try this experiment. Imagine you are about to have your favourite snack. Maybe it's mature cheddar cheese on a cracker with some really tangy pickle. Maybe it's an onion bhaji. Maybe it's a crisp, juicy apple. Whatever it is, just anticipate it for a moment.

Did your mouth water a little? I'm sure it did. That means you caused a response from your autonomic nervous system simply by imagining something. That's the part of your nervous system that, normally acting below the level of consciousness, controls such things as heart rate, respiration rate, and digestion. Just think about it for a moment. You, as it were, 'tricked' your autonomic nervous system by using visualization.

These experiments are not trivial. They establish that you have a certain mental ability to regulate pain, known as Mind Controlled Analgesia (MCA). And like any ability it can be improved.

In Chapter 1 I made the claim that there was a close connection between emotional pain and physical pain, especially chronic physical pain. Where, you may be asking, is the evidence? In fact, there's a great deal. A study of 75 women with fibromyalgia found that 57 per cent had a history of sexual or physical abuse and, compared with non-abused sufferers, they had more health problems and needed more medication. A study at the University of Alabama looked at 13 women with gastroesophageal reflux disease (GERD), 26 with noncardiac chest pain (NCCP) and 11 with irritable bowel syndrome (IBS). It transpired that 92 per cent of those with GERD and 82 per cent of those with IBS had suffered sexual or physical abuse. Abused patients had a lower pain threshold than non-abused patients and, in addition, they were more likely to have other additional pain syndromes. Yet another study, by the University of New Brunswick Faculty of Nursing, looked at 292 women who had separated from abusive partners and found that more than one-third suffered high disability pain and that 43.2 per cent specifically had swollen or painful joints. And there have been many other studies that have come up with similar results.

If it's true that there's this connection between emotional pain and physical pain then we'd expect emotional people to suffer pain more keenly than the less emotional. And that's exactly what we do see. In general, women are more emotional than men and a study led by Dr Ed Keogh, a psychologist at the Pain Management Unit at Bath University, found that women do have a lower pain threshold than men, and experience pain more frequently than men in more areas of their bodies.

The 'female' hormone oestrogen could have something to do with it because it's known, for example, that women's pain thresholds vary during the menstrual cycle. But there is another factor at work, too. The Bath University scientists concluded that women respond to pain in a more emotional way than men and consequently find it harder to bear. That ties in with research at Leeds Metropolitan University which concluded that, because of the male need to appear macho, men were less likely to admit to pain and tried harder to master it.

It's vitally important that you understand and accept this principle. Having, say, fibromyalgia does not mean that you were abused in some way in the past. But if you were abused then your chance of having fibromyalgia or several other painful conditions increases. If you do have an emotionally induced pain condition, or a painful condition exacerbated by your emotional state, then treatment must involve your mind. It's also the case that chronic pain causes physical changes in the structure of the brain and those changes have to be reversed somehow. The way is through Mind Controlled Analgesia.

Here's a little test of your MCA abilities and attitudes right now.

Diagnostic test

Select the answer that most closely represents your situation.

1 Has a physical cause for your pain been clearly identified?

  a No
  b Yes

2 Are you susceptible to hypnosis?

  a Yes
  b No

3 Hypnosis is:

  a Something that really works
  b Just a load of stage magic – it isn't real

4 My pain:

  a Is bad at times but there are things that help
  b Never gets less – nothing ever seems to help

5 Pain relief:

  a Is something in which I must play my part – it can't all be left to the medical profession
  b Is not something within my control – I just have to have faith in the medical profession

6 My pain:

  a Is not going to stop me doing the things I want
  b Prevents me doing anything

7 When the pain is bad:

  a I do my best to carry on
  b I get myself all cosy and wait for it to pass

8 I believe pain is:

   a A sign that I need to mobilize myself more efficiently
   b A signal that I should cease physical activities

9 My pain:

   a Is something I sometimes forget when I'm distracted
   b Is always on my mind

10 I take pain medication:

   a At regular intervals
   b When the pain comes on

▶ **Your score**

▶ If you answered mostly 'a' you're someone who is already very open to psychological methods of pain control. You're a fighter and you're willing to try everything to beat the problem.

▶ If you answered mostly 'b' you're probably sceptical about psychological methods and prefer to leave things to the doctors. But that doesn't mean psychological methods can't work for you, if you'll just give them a chance.

Neuro-Linguistic Programming (NLP)

Milton H Erickson (1901–1980) contracted polio at the age of 17 and was severely paralysed. Lying in bed day after day his main entertainment was to observe the interactions of his eight siblings. His parents had been told he would die but Erickson was a man of extraordinary willpower. He gradually recovered the use of his voice and his arms and, partially, his legs, setting off alone on a thousand mile canoe trip, by the end of which he was able to walk with a cane.

Polio was an experience that gave him an unrivalled insight into the mind–body connection, both by observing others and observing himself, and, after studying medicine and psychology, he began to develop his own system of hypnotherapy. His astonishing results attracted the attention of, among many others, two young men called John Grinder and Richard Bandler. The duo very carefully studied – or, as they called it, 'modelled' – Erickson's methods to discover exactly what he did, what worked and what didn't. From that they developed their own system of therapy which they called Neuro-Linguistic Programming (NLP).

OVERLOADING AND DISTRACTION

Overloading and distraction are two simple NLP techniques. It's fairly well established that the conscious mind can only handle seven items (plus or minus two) at any time. Overloading the brain therefore means something has to be ignored and, with a bit of luck, it will be the pain. Distraction works in a similar way but uses one very powerful stimulus instead of several lesser ones.

In fact, we're probably all familiar with this kind of phenomenon, receiving an injury but being completely unaware of it at the time because we're preoccupied by a task or by, say, the need to escape a fire or a crash or something like that.

Try it now

Find yourself a task that is absolutely riveting and that requires various kinds of mental activity. What you choose will obviously depend very much on your personality. A game such as poker can be good because it involves all sorts of things such as remembering cards, reading the body language of the other players, taking conscious control of your own body language, calculating how much to bet and, of course, interacting socially. If you're alone you might like to try playing a computer game. If you have sufficient mobility try exercising (walking, jogging or whatever) while listening to music and keeping your heart rate within a particular range. Whatever you're doing, always look for ways to create extra inputs and extra intensity so there's less room for pain signals.

VISUALIZATION

We all use visualization every day but most of us don't use it very effectively. Grinder and Bandler saw that it had a lot more potential and looked to the cinema for inspiration.

Let's take a woman who needs an operation and is already anticipating the pain. When we're afraid of things we tend to imagine them *big*. So when this woman visualizes the opening in her abdomen she has it completely filling her 'screen'. The image is all in disturbing shades of red. The beeping of the heart monitor is as loud as a burglar alarm. She smells the antiseptic.

These kinds of qualities of a mental image – size, colour, loudness, and so on – are known in NLP as 'submodalities'. The concept behind NLP visualization is that instead of the way you feel creating the submodalities, you deliberately create the submodalities that will make you feel the way you would prefer to be. In other words, instead of seeing the opening full screen you reduce the size. Instead of the image being in shades of red you introduce creams and pastel blue. The bleeping of the heart monitor becomes a gentle, regular, almost meditative sound. And the smell of antiseptic is replaced by the smell of a favourite perfume.

Most people have probably never given a thought to the submodalities of their internal cinema. So, if that includes you, here's a little exercise.

Try it now

Lie down somewhere comfortable and have a notebook and pen handy.

Call up an image of a person you really love. Write down in your notebook the submodalities. For example, is the image in colour or in black and white? Is it vivid or faint? Is it large or small? Is it central or to one side? Can you hear music?

Next think about your pain. If you had to convey to someone what it was like what would you say? That it was like being devoured by ants? Like being stabbed with a sword? Like being burnt by flames? Again write down the submodalities.

Here are some possibilities that may help you.

Visual qualities (submodalities)
* Colour or black and white
* Large or small
* Near or far

* Bright or dull
* Moving or still
* Clear or blurred

Audio qualities (submodalities)
* Loud or soft
* High pitched or low pitched
* Clear or muffled
* Near or far
* Pleasant or unpleasant

Qualities of feelings (kinaesthetic submodalities)
* Heavy or light
* Rough or smooth
* Hot or cold
* Constant or intermittent
* Strong or weak
* Moving or still
* Intense or faint
* Sharp or dull
* Increasing or decreasing heart rate
* Faster or slower breathing rate.

Once you've got the hang of identifying submodalities the next step is to begin manipulating them deliberately.

 Try it now

In your imagination create a short movie that shows your pain diminishing. One idea, often used in NLP, is to visualize your pain being shut away in a box. Gradually you crush the box, one side at a time, turning it round and round, until it's so small you can toss it far away. Another idea is to visualize the painful area as being a particular colour while normal flesh is a different colour. The painful area is slowly painted with a soothing liquid which changes its colour to that of normal flesh. Whatever mental movie you select, try the following manipulations to see how they change the impact of the film.

* See the scene through your own eyes.
* Switch 'cameras' to see the scene from another person's viewpoint.

* Make a split screen and show different images side by side.
* Run a section in slow motion.
* Show a series of stills.
* Play some music.
* Play some completely different music.
* Use soft focus.
* Introduce a voiceover.
* Zoom in for a close-up.
* Change the colour scheme.
* Shrink the image to half the screen then a quarter then an eighth.

Don't worry if you can't actually see an image very clearly or for very long. That's how it is for most people. But the more you practise the better you'll get at it.

Each time you manipulate the image ask yourself what effect it has on you. How does it impact your emotions? For example, you might feel:
* More/less confident
* More/less involved
* More/less happy
* More/less afraid
* More/less in pain

Remember this

Make time to carry out these experiments in submodalities every day. See if you can improve your ability to visualize. If you have to commute by train regularly this is a good way of creatively passing the journey.

THE CIRCLE OF EASE

The Circle of Confidence is a standard NLP technique for transferring confidence from a situation in which you feel mastery to a situation in which you feel inadequate. Here the technique has been adapted for pain relief. It's called *The Circle of Ease*.

Try it now

Step 1. Think back to a specific time when, although you had your pain, you were able to handle it much more easily than now. Possibly you were able to ignore it completely. Perhaps there was a special, very happy occasion when the strength of your emotions blotted everything else out.

Step 2. Relive that time, seeing and hearing everything in as much detail as possible. Particularly notice how at ease you looked.

Step 3. Imagine a circle on the floor. Take the ease you felt back then and pour it into the circle. Immediately the circle takes on a colour – the colour that, to you, is the colour of being at ease. Add in some music that's uplifting to you – perhaps the *Chariots of Fire* theme by Vangelis.

Step 4. Are there any other qualities you had back then which could help you overcome pain now? Maybe confidence? Maybe determination? Maybe optimism? If so, repeat the procedure, also pouring those qualities into your circle.

Step 5. When you have everything you need in *The Circle of Ease*, step into it and visualize all those qualities rising up from the floor, permeating and enveloping you like steam in a Turkish bath, easing your pain away.

Step 6. From now on you will always be enveloped in that comforting, soothing sense of ease. Your *Circle* will move with you. But you may need to top it up from time to time by running through Steps 1–5 again.

STRESS AND PAIN

It's a fact that the more stressed you are, the more pain you feel. Here's one NLP method for inducing relaxation and combating stress, using a technique known as 'anchoring'.

An anchor in NLP is something that causes an automatic response. For example, if you're driving a car and you see brake lights go on ahead of you so, without even thinking, you take your foot off the accelerator and move it to the brake pedal. In this instance, brake lights ahead are the anchor and the action of getting ready to brake is the automatic response.

Try it now

Step 1. Recall a time when you felt *incredibly* relaxed. Fully experience that sense of relaxation. Feel, see, hear, smell and taste the elements that made you that way. Identify the submodalities for relaxation.

Step 2. Create a break state by saying your telephone number backwards.

Step 3. Re-experience the relaxation you created in Step 1. Take the submodalities for relaxation and adjust them until you're approaching the optimum level but not quite there. At that very moment do the following:

* Bring your hand up to your face so you can see it.
* Stroke the sides of your face between your thumb and forefinger.
* Whisper the word 'relax' to yourself.

Those three actions are your anchors. Note that one is visual (seeing your hand), one is kinaesthetic (feeling your fingers stroking your face) and one is audible (hearing the word 'relax'). You can choose three other anchors if you wish but you should always have one in each category.

Step 4. Create a break state by saying your telephone number backwards.

Step 5. Repeat Step 3 several times. On each occasion try to improve the whole thing so that you feel more and more relaxed and your anchor-setting technique gets better and better.

Step 6. Fire your anchors – that's to say, repeat the three actions from Step 3. If you feel relaxed as a result then the procedure has worked. Your three anchors are now automatically inducing a state of relaxation.

Step 7. Think of future potentially distressing situations in which you would like to feel more at ease. As you do so, fire your anchors. This will set things up for you so that when those situations come about you'll already be primed to become relaxed.

Step 8. Live life and whenever you encounter stressful situations for real, fire your anchors. The more often you repeat the procedure and the more often you use the anchors the more powerful the effect will be.

FEAR AND PAIN

It sometimes happens that chronic pain is a response to a phobia. The unconscious mind creates the pain to prevent you ever having to confront the thing you're afraid of. Let's say, for example, that you have a phobia about leaving the house (agoraphobia). In that case, your unconscious might create pain in your legs so you have a 'genuine excuse' not to go out.

NLP has a technique for dealing with phobia, *provided the phobia was acquired during a particular incident.* If you can cure the phobia the associated pain should go away. It's known as the *Fast Phobia Technique*.

Try it now

Step 1. Imagine that you're in a cinema. In this cinema you're going to be in as many as three places at once – appearing in the film, watching it as a customer and working as the projectionist, all at the same time. (That's the wonderful thing about the imagination – you can do anything you like.)

Step 2. Be a customer sitting in the cinema, watching a still black and white image of yourself on the screen the moment *before* you experienced this fear for the very first time. (If you can't remember when you first had the fear, instead use an image of the moment before you experienced the fear the most intensely.)

Step 3. Now you're going to become the projectionist sitting in the projection booth. As the projectionist you can now see yourself in the cinema as well as the image on screen.

Step 4. Still as the projectionist you run the black and white movie of the frightening situation. You see everything but it means almost nothing to you because you're just a projectionist, sitting in the safety of your projection booth. When you get to the end of the movie, where the person in the film (you) is safe again, you stop the projector and freeze frame.

Step 5. This is where things get really tricky. You have to leave the projection booth and step into the still picture on the screen. It now turns to full colour and as it does so the movie runs backwards very quickly. In other words, everyone walks backwards and talks backwards. So it should all look and sound quite funny and to underline how laughable it is you need to have a film score of comical music (the sort of thing you might hear at the circus). Hearing this music and the backwards voices and seeing the ridiculous movements, *laugh*.

Step 6. Repeat the backwards film sequence several more times, getting faster and faster each time.

Richard Bandler claims he's never failed with this technique. But you don't have the experience of Richard Bandler so you may have to be prepared to carry out the procedure a few times. If, after completing the six steps, the object of your fear still scores a three or higher on a scale of one to ten, then repeat the procedure. If you rate it from zero to two then go out in the real world and see what happens.

Key idea

Richard Bandler has written in his book *Get the Life You Want* that after running the technique readers should get up from their chairs 'and test it, and test it, and test it' and that 'bit by bit' the phobia will disappear.

Case study

At the time of writing you can see Richard Bandler in action on YouTube in a two-part video called *The Hypnotist*. In this he treats a woman distressed by what she tells him is a phobia about flying brought on by a hijacking 27 years earlier. (In fact, Bandler diagnoses her not as suffering from a phobia but from panic attacks brought on by any enclosed environment and, indeed, that proves to be the case.)

Bandler augments the *Fast Phobia Technique* with hypnosis and then takes her out for desensitization by gradual exposure. He has her ride in a lift with other people, a situation she normally finds overwhelming. From there he takes her to a cinema. The final test is to take a flight. During this the patient again suffers a panic attack but overcomes it.

So it was a success for NLP but *not* an instant success and, realistically, you shouldn't expect to do better on yourself than Richard Bandler did.

SIX STEP REFRAMING

Pain is a signal that something is wrong. Once you know something is wrong and are taking action to deal with it the pain is redundant. In an ideal world it would go away. But the body is not quite that sophisticated.

Developed by John Grinder, *Six Step Reframing* is a technique in which you'll speak to your unconscious as if it's a separate person and ask it to turn the pain off. At first *Six Step Reframing* may well strike you as a little wacky. However, once you try it you'll fairly soon get used to 'talking to yourself' and think of it as normal.

Step 1. Identify the pain.

Step 2. You now need to get in touch with your unconscious. This is something easily achieved by a trained hypnotherapist. Doing it on your own is a bit more tricky. Grinder suggests asking something like: 'Will you, my unconscious, communicate with me?' You must then wait passively with your attention focused on your body for a signal from your unconscious. If you receive a signal, touch the area of your body where the signal occurred and say, 'Thank you'. To check you then ask: 'If the signal just offered means yes, please repeat it.' You now need to validate the repeated signal. Asking your unconscious to remain inactive, you now try to reproduce the signal consciously. If you can then the possibility exists that the signal wasn't a genuine signal from the unconscious and you'll need to repeat the process until you have an authentic involuntary signal. Examples of the kinds of signals your unconscious could give you that you couldn't very easily reproduce consciously include:

- Tingling down the back of your neck or spine

- Fluttering or pulsating of a muscle

- A localized hot or tickling sensation

- A localized numbness

Step 3. Ask your unconscious: 'What is the positive intention behind the creation of pain in my leg (or wherever it is)?' Let's assume you get the answer, 'To prevent you damaging it any further.'

Step 4. Having discovered the positive intention you now need to generate a set of alternatives as good or better than the pain at satisfying that positive intention. You might say something like this to your unconscious: 'I know the leg is broken and it's now in plaster. There's no need for the pain. Please develop an alternative to pain that will nevertheless still satisfy the positive intention. When you have completed the task give me a signal.'

Step 5. Your unconscious might now say something like this: 'I know you. If there's no pain you'll be running around as if there's nothing wrong. I'll only stop the pain if you agree to rest, relax and get help around the home.' Get your unconscious to accept responsibility for implementing the new behaviours. For example, you might ask: 'Will you, my unconscious mind, take responsibility for making sure the new behaviours are followed?'

Step 6. Ask your unconscious to make sure the changes it makes will not be the cause of new problems for you or for those around you.

Self-hypnosis

In April 1845, Dr James Esdaile was operating on a man with a swollen testicle. The procedure was particularly painful and this was two years before the Scottish obstetrician James Young Simpson discovered the anaesthetic qualities of chloroform. Dr Esdaile turned to his assistant and asked if he knew anything about Mesmerism, the name then used for what we now call hypnotism.

'I have a great mind to try it on this man,' said Dr Esdaile, 'but as I never saw it practised, and know it only from reading, I shall probably not succeed.'

He did try it, he did succeed and he went on to complete many more operations using hypnosis. And had it not been for James Young Simpson, hypnosis might well be the standard form of anaesthesia today.

You can't actually be hypnotized by someone else. You can go to see a hypnotherapist and be led by that person into trance. But the hypnotherapist can't *make* you hypnotized. All hypnosis is actually self-hypnosis. Which means you can very effectively use self-hypnosis at home for pain relief.

What is hypnosis? Derren Brown, the TV mentalist says he doesn't know what hypnotism really is himself. What we can say for sure is that it's an altered state of consciousness or, more specifically, a state of consciousness that's different to what we consider to be our normal waking state. In other words, a trance.

In fact, we all go into trances every day. When you're totally absorbed in a book or a newspaper and unaware of the things going on around you you're in a trance. It's as simple as that. When you swing a golf club or throw a dart and get almost exactly the result you want you're in a trance. When you're making love with your partner you're in a trance.

Key idea

Floating above the ground rigid as a board is stage magic and has nothing to do with hypnosis. Real hypnosis can achieve dramatic results but it can't overturn the laws of physics nor bring about complete pain relief in a single session. In many cases, professional hypnotherapists might recommend ten to fourteen weekly one-to-one sessions with daily home sessions on CDs in between. That's something like 100 sessions. As an amateur at self-hypnosis you should expect to do as much. Of course, you can expect a degree of pain relief much sooner but the maximum effect will take time.

Try it now

Step 1. Get yourself comfortable in a place you won't be disturbed. It's not a good idea to lie on the bed because you might fall asleep. But you could sit up on the bed supported by pillows, or arrange yourself in a comfy chair.

Step 2. Decide the length of time you wish to spend in self-hypnosis. Initially I'd suggest 10 minutes. That should give you enough time to achieve a deep state of trance without feeling anxiety about 'wasting' time or needing to get on with something else. As you get used to self-hypnosis you can vary the time. So, having got comfortable, you should say something like this: 'I am now going to hypnotize myself for 10 minutes'. You might like to append the actual time by adding '...which means I will come out of self-hypnosis at 19.30 (or whatever)'.

Step 3. This is a key step because it's where you state the purpose of your hypnosis. Here we're concerned with pain relief, but you could also use the technique to make you feel, say, more confident or more relaxed or more determined. The exact words aren't important. Something along these lines will do fine:

✳ I am entering into a state of self-hypnosis so that I can hand over to my unconscious mind the task of reducing the pain in my back.

✳ I am entering into a trance for the purpose of allowing my unconscious mind to make the adjustments that will reduce my sensation of pain.

✱ I am entering into a trance for the purpose of allowing my unconscious mind to correct an error in my nervous system. Pain is a signal that something is wrong. I have received that message and everything that could be done is being done so there's no point now in continuing the pain.

✱ I am entering into a trance so that I can hand over to my unconscious mind the task of separating, for a while, the real me from my body. I will leave my body here in bed and the real me will go and watch television.

Whatever you say, make sure it includes the message that you are inviting your *unconscious* to deal with the matter.

Step 4. State how you want to feel when you come out of your trance. For example, you might say, '...and as I come out of my trance I will feel happy, light and optimistic'. Or if you're practising self-hypnosis last thing at night you might say, '...and as I come out of my trance I will feel ready to enjoy a blissful night's sleep.' Why not say that as you come out of trance you'll no longer feel pain? The problem is that by searching to see if the pain is still there you'll focus on it and unwittingly increase it again.

Step 5. This is the actual process of self-hypnosis. Basically you're going to engage in turn your three main representational systems (sight, hearing, touch) to bring the trance about. In the first part of the process you will be noting things you can actually see, hear and feel *in the room where you are*. In the second part you will be noting things you can see, hear and feel *in an imaginary scene*.

Below is a diagram that represents the whole process. In the diagram, V = Visual System, A = Auditory System, and K = Kinaesthetic System.

V	V	V
A	A	A
K	K	K
V	V	
A	A	
K	K	
V		
A		
K		
(External)		

- -

```
V
A
K
V               V
A               A
K               K
V               V               V
A               A               A
K               K               K
```

In this process, some people talk to themselves internally but I recommend that *you say everything out loud*. For that reason you'll want to be in a private place. You might imagine that you'd 'wake' yourself up but, in fact, the sound of your own voice, done the right way, will intensify the effect. (If, however, speaking out loud doesn't work for you then by all means speak internally.)

(a) From your comfortable position look at some small thing in the room in front of you and say out loud what you are looking at. Choose things you can see without moving your head. For example, 'I am looking at the door handle'. Then, without rushing, focus on another small item. For example, 'I am now looking at a glass of water on the table.' Then move on to a third item. For example, 'I am looking at the light switch'. When you have your three visual references, move on to (b).

(b) Switch attention to sounds and, in the same way, note one after another until you have three, each time saying out loud what you're hearing. Then move on to (c).

(c) Note things that you can feel with your body. For example, you might say, 'I can feel the seat pressing against my buttocks.' When you have your three, move on.

(d) Now repeat steps (a) to (c) but with only two items for each sense, that's to say, two images, two sounds and two feelings. They must be *different* from the ones you used before. *Speak a little more slowly*.

(e) Again repeat steps (a) to (c) but with only one item per sense, that's to say, one image, one sound and one feeling.

Again, they must be *different* from any that have gone before. *Speak even more slowly.*

(f) Close your eyes, if they're not already closed, and think of a happy scene in which you are free of pain. To keep things simple, make it a still picture. It might, for example, be you with a group of friends playing with a ball on the beach on a sunny day. It might be you and your partner throwing sticks for your dog. It might be you floating serenely in a warm bath.

(g) Using this imagined scene, go through the same process you already used for the real scene, but beginning with just one example of each of the three senses, that is, one image, one sound and one feeling. When you've done that, increase to two examples and then three. (Three is usually enough, but if you've stipulated a lengthy session you may need to continue with your fantasy scene by going on to name four images, sounds and feelings, or five or even more.) Remember, each example must be *different*. You'll probably find you're automatically speaking very slowly now but, if not, make a point of *slowing your voice down more and more.*

(h) After the allotted time you should begin to come out of trance automatically. But it may help to announce, 'I'll count to three and when I reach three I'll be (whatever you said in Step 4)'. Don't worry about getting 'stuck' in a trance. That won't happen. You may feel a little woozy for a while. If so, don't drive a car or do anything demanding until you're sure you're okay to do so.

Key idea

In his fifties, Milton Erickson developed post-polio syndrome which caused muscle weakness and severe pain. He used self-hypnosis to keep the pain under control but even he, one of the most successful hypnotherapists of all time, had to repeat it every day. As he explained: 'It usually takes me an hour after I awaken to get all the pain out.' One session of self-hypnosis should help but, like Milton Erickson, be ready to 'top up' regularly.

BREAKTHROUGH

If you've succeeded in at least one of the NLP techniques and also achieved a state of self-hypnosis you've made a breakthrough and are ready to move on to the next chapter. If none of the techniques in this chapter has achieved anything for you, try them again. Even if your pain has an entirely physical cause these techniques should reduce your perception of pain.

Focus points

✻ We all have the ability to decrease our sensitivity to pain – as has been proven many, many times in emergency situations as well as everyday life.

✻ NLP has several techniques for reducing the perception of pain, including distraction, overloading and visualization.

✻ NLP can combat the stress that heightens pain.

✻ The unconscious can sometimes create pain to protect you from something you fear.

✻ You can directly engage your unconscious to reduce pain through Six Step Reframing and self-hypnosis.

Next step

In the next chapter we'll be looking at more techniques of Mind Controlled Analgesia, especially cognitive therapy (CT) which has a well-established track record. The more of these psychological tools you have at your disposal the more likely you are to find one that really suits you. You'll also be learning about the value of support groups.

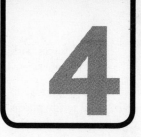

More Mind Controlled Analgesia

In this chapter you will learn:

▶ *more techniques of Mind Controlled Analgesia (MCA)*

▶ *how your brain may be the cause of your problems*

▶ *how cognitive behavioural therapy (CBT) can help*

▶ *how to detach from pain.*

> Natural forces within us are the true healers of disease.
> Hippocrates, Greek physician (c.460 BCE – c.370 BCE)

In the last chapter we looked at Neuro-Linguistic Programming (NLP) and self-hypnosis as ways of reducing pain. In this chapter we're going to be looking at some other methods of Mind Controlled Analgesia (MCA). Once you've read and absorbed both chapters you'll have a pretty complete toolbox of self-help psychological approaches.

Let me once again state that a psychological approach to pain relief in no way implies that your pain isn't real. As we saw in Chapter 1, the pain system works something like a burglar alarm. To stop it going off we could interfere with the sensors or we could interfere with the central computer. The brain is the central computer. I repeat that modern scanning techniques have revealed that chronic pain causes alterations in the structure of the brain. To beat chronic pain those alterations need to be reversed.

First of all, let's see how well the MCA techniques in this chapter are likely to work for you.

? Diagnostic test

1 In the past year have you suffered separation, divorce or the death of your partner?

2 In the past year have you married or become reconciled with a former partner?

3 In the past year have you lost your job or retired?

4 In the past year have you suffered the death of someone close?

5 In the past year have you suffered a major illness or injury or been in prison?

6 Do you anger easily or sometimes feel irritable without knowing why?

7 Do you think your life now is stressful?

8 Do you know or have reason to believe you were abused, or had other serious problems, as a child?

9 Do you feel unfairly victimized by your pain or that you're less of a person because you're in pain?

10 Do you think about your pain often?

▶ **Your score**

Questions 1 – 5 cover what are generally considered to be the top ten stressors in anybody's life. The more of them to which you answered 'yes' the more likely you are to suffer physical pain.

Questions 6 and 7 cover the stress you're under now. Again, if you answered 'yes' to either or both you're liable to have a heightened pain response.

The significance of question 8 is that sufferers of a wide range of painful conditions, including fibromyalgia and irritable bowel syndrome, are significantly more likely than average to have experienced childhood trauma. If that should be your case, treating the pain involves dealing with those memories, both conscious and unconscious.

Questions 9 and 10 cover your attitude to pain. If you answered 'yes' to either or both then a new way of looking at your situation may be helpful.

In general, then, the more you answered 'yes' the more MCA is likely to work for you.

Cognitive behavioural therapy (CBT)

Various trials have shown that a technique known as cognitive behavioural therapy (CBT):

▶ Reduces pain

▶ Improves mood and combats pain-related depression

▶ Helps sufferers to cope with pain

▶ Increases physical activity

The behavioural aspects (breathing techniques, relaxation exercises, stress management, and so on) are dealt with elsewhere in the book. Here we'll concentrate on the cognitive (thinking) aspect.

Cognitive therapy (CT) was pioneered in the 1960s by Dr Aaron Beck at the University of Pennsylvania School of Medicine. Dr Beck noticed that most of the patients who came to him with depression had views of themselves and their lives that were out of step with reality. Successful professional people would tell him they were failures. Men with warm, supportive families would say nobody loved them. Women with happy, well-adjusted children would say they were awful mothers. Dr Beck realized it wasn't reality that was causing depression but the way people thought about reality. And the same principle applies to pain. If your thoughts about your pain are unduly pessimistic and unhelpful so you'll feel the pain more keenly and be less likely to lead a fulfilling life.

Here are some thoughts you might have concerning your pain:

▶ Other people don't suffer pain like this – it's so unfair.

▶ Since I'm not perfectly free from pain this treatment is no good.

▶ This is the worst pain anybody has ever experienced.

▶ I'm an invalid.

▶ I'm sure this pain means I'm going to die.

Let's look at these in detail.

OTHER PEOPLE DON'T SUFFER PAIN LIKE THIS – IT'S SO UNFAIR

This is an unhelpful way of thinking known as 'comparing'. The problem is that we all naturally tend to compare with people who seem to be better off, people who are richer, more attractive, fitter – and pain free. Believing that you're alone, and that you've somehow been singled out, makes you feel all the more distressed which, in turn, increases your sensation of pain.

▶ The solution

Compare yourself instead with the one-fifth of the world's population who suffer chronic pain – many of them without access to effective painkillers. And the figure rises to one-third among the elderly. In addition, everyone suffers from acute pain from time to time. So you're definitely not alone in suffering pain and you haven't been unfairly singled out. It may help you to join a support group where you can exchange experiences and information and receive encouragement from others who are in the same boat. Feeling victimized is only going to increase your physical and emotional pain. Tell yourself this: 'I'm one out of millions of people suffering pain but I'm one of the fortunate ones because I have access to the most advanced treatments on the planet.'

SINCE I'M NOT PERFECTLY FREE FROM PAIN THIS TREATMENT IS NO GOOD

This statement combines two cognitive errors. One is the search for perfection and the other is what's known as 'black and white' thinking. Instead of seeing your treatment as substantially successful you regard it as totally ineffective. As a result, you lose the positive psychological element that is always a component in a successful outcome.

▶ The solution

Perfection just doesn't exist. Nothing and no one is perfect. Just look around you. Couldn't you improve on everything you see? And pain treatments are no different. They can always be faster, more effective, freer from side effects. Don't focus on the shortcomings. Focus instead on the benefits. And certainly don't indulge in the black and white thinking that says if something doesn't work perfectly it's no good at all. Black and white thinking is very convenient mental shorthand. Either a medicament is great or it's useless. Either a doctor is brilliant or she's hopeless. Either you're free of pain or you're in agony. But real life isn't actually like that. Real life is in shades of grey. Medicaments may only work to a degree, doctors all make mistakes, and pain is usually in the middle range and variable. Whilst staying alive to the possibility that there may be better treatments, accept the idea that no treatment is perfect. (We'll be looking at acceptance in more detail in a moment.)

THIS IS THE WORST PAIN ANYBODY HAS EVER EXPERIENCED

This is an example of exaggeration. Here are some others. 'I can't do anything because of this pain.' 'Nothing ever reduces my pain.' 'This pain has taken control of my life.' We all exaggerate. Often it's harmless fun, as when telling friends about the fish that got away or the compliment we received. But when you exaggerate to yourself about your degree of pain and the consequences it has for your life then you're talking yourself into a negative state that can only make things worse.

▶ The solution

One way of getting a more accurate handle on things is to keep a diary. In it record the times you feel little or no pain. And record the things you're able to do during those pain-free or low-pain episodes. When you're feeling despondent take a look at what you've written. You'll probably be surprised at how much you've been able to accomplish and how often you've felt happy.

I'M AN INVALID

The problem with labels is that they tend to stick, permanently. Once you start to think of yourself as 'an invalid' or some such label so you build a mental structure accordingly. And by acting the part of 'an invalid' so you cause other people to respond to you that way, too. They won't expect you to join in normal activities with them. They'll perhaps treat you as 'second class'. None of that is helpful in developing an optimistic outlook.

▶ The solution

Stop thinking of yourself as 'an invalid' or anything like that. Instead, label yourself by your many positive qualities. Think of yourself as 'the musician', 'the lover', 'the person getting better' or whatever more favourable title fits.

I'M SURE THIS PAIN MEANS I'M GOING TO DIE

This is an example of 'jumping to negative conclusions'. You hear two nurses whispering and assume they're saying something worrying about you. You go for tests and feel sure the results will be the worst possible. You have a pain and conclude it's a sign of something fatal.

▶ The solution

Some of the worst pains are associated with conditions that are far from life threatening. Kidney stones can be agonizing, hiatus hernia can resemble a massive heart attack, and migraine can render the strongest men incapable of movement or even speech. Think back to all the times in your life that you've made negative predictions. How many of them turned out to be true? Let's find out. Keep a little notebook with you for one day and every time you make a negative prediction about anything (she'll be late, I'll never manage this, something dreadful is wrong) write it down. At bedtime do the sums. You'll probably find that most things turn out far better than your forecast.

Case study

'I was with a group of riders when the horses were spooked and several people got thrown off. One young woman said her back had been injured and I immediately drove her to a nearby hospital. While the woman was lying on a trolley, waiting for a doctor to come, her pain was intensifying. She felt sure her back was broken, that only immediate action could save her from paralysis, and begged me to get help for her urgently. She seemed to be in agony. I did my best to hurry things but it was still about a quarter of an hour – which seemed much longer – before a doctor arrived. He was middle-aged and had an authoritative manner. He touched the woman here and there, asking, "Can you feel that?" She could. "I want you to sit up and touch your calves," he said. "I'll support you with my hand." She did. "That's fine," he said. "There's nothing wrong." At these words the woman brightened, got off the trolley and happily walked to the car. As for me, I felt a bit stupid.' John (35)

Acceptance and Commitment Therapy plus mindfulness

Acceptance and Commitment Therapy (ACT) is a relatively new name but an approach that goes back a long way. It's mostly used in psychotherapy for the treatment of depression but the same principles can be used for the control of pain. Mindfulness is often taught as a discipline on its own but I'll be including it here as a technique within ACT.

ACCEPTANCE

ACT goes back to the Buddha (Siddhartha Gautama) if not before. The Buddha it was who spent 49 days meditating under a tree, seeking to know why people suffered and what could be done about it. His message was simple. Suffering can be ended by detaching.

While staying at the Anathapindaka monastery at Savatthi, the Buddha is said to have explained it to his son Rahula in the following terms: 'All material forms, past, present, or future, within or without, gross or subtle, base or fine, far or near, all should be viewed with full understanding, with the thought: "This is not mine, this is not I, this is not my soul".'

When it comes to physical pain, then, your aim is to detach from it. To notice it and accept it without reacting to it. The pain is in your body but your body isn't really you. That may seem a bizarre concept at first. But ask yourself this: 'If I lost a limb would I still be me?' No doubt you'd answer 'yes'. So 'you' seem to be something linked to but nevertheless separate from your body.

Remember this

Acceptance can seem a pretty pathetic response to pain (or any of life's problems). But it doesn't mean that you do nothing at all to help yourself. (That's where the commitment bit comes in, as we'll see in a moment.) What it does mean is that you don't make your emotional state (and therefore your pain) worse by feeling bitter and negative.

Try it now

Recall an upsetting thought you sometimes have about your pain, such as 'I can never enjoy myself because of this pain' or 'I'm a rotten parent because of this pain'. Note how that makes you feel. Now try putting these words in front: 'I'm having the thought that...' Now how do you feel?

The idea is to help you realize that a thought is just a thought. It isn't the thing itself and it may not be an accurate assessment anyway.

Another technique is to take a negative phrase that bothers you (such as 'Everyone is fed up with me because of my pain') and try to see the actual words in different ways. Again the idea is to help you realize that these are just words not reality. So visualize the words in front of you and try changing the colour, the size, the typeface and the position. Then set fire to them or pour acid over them and watch them disappear. You see, they have no substance at all.

MINDFULNESS

All day long thoughts are coming into your head. Some are concerned with what you're doing right now but others – usually the majority – will consist of memories, fantasies, deductions, visualizations of the future, and so on. Some of those thoughts may be enjoyable but many of them will be unpleasant. And those unpleasant thoughts can make you feel embarrassed, anxious, fearful, low, and even depressed. In turn, those emotions can exacerbate pain and cause other physical problems.

When you're actually in pain the situation is worse. Quite naturally you worry about the cause of the pain, wonder what the future will hold, and feel upset or angry about the unfairness of it.

When all of that is going on in your mind you hardly notice what's going on around you. You miss out on all the things that used to give you pleasure – the sun on your skin, a beautiful view, music, the conversation of friends, or whatever it might be. The idea of mindfulness is to reverse your mental state. Instead of your pain crowding out everything else, you use everything else to crowd out your pain. In other words, you live much more in the moment.

Think about the worst mistake you ever made in your life, the worst thing you've ever done, or the worst few minutes you've ever experienced. Really relive that incident. See the whole ghastly thing. Now how do you feel? Perhaps a tightening across the chest? Maybe butterflies in the stomach? Possibly a beating in one or other temple? And yet you were only *thinking* about something. It wasn't real. That shows how powerful your imagination is and how much damage it can do. That's why you have to get it under control.

Of course, no one is saying you should completely deny yourself the pleasure of reliving joyful past events, of looking forward to future events, or of creating gorgeous fantasies. In fact, thinking about something pleasurable activates the mesolimbic dopamine system in the brain almost as much as actually doing the thing. So carry on with your happy recollections, projections and daydreams – the day you fell in love, a forthcoming holiday, perhaps an exciting fantasy about yourself and someone you're attracted to. But these kinds of thoughts should be a much smaller percentage of your mental life than they probably are now. And when it comes to upsetting thoughts about your pain, use the technique of focusing on the present to reduce them to almost nothing.

Try it now

Find something to drink (it could be a glass of wine, a cup of tea or even water). Also find something simple to eat (for example, a few olives, a piece of bread, or an apple). Take a gulp of whatever you're drinking and swallow it immediately. Similarly, take a bite of your snack and swallow it at once. After a pause, again take a mouthful of your drink but this time roll it around your tongue, savour it, try to describe the flavour or flavours, and let it trickle only a little at a time down your throat. Similarly, take a bite of your snack, chew it carefully, move it around your mouth, identify the flavour or flavours, and only then swallow it. This is the difference between non-mindfulness and mindfulness. Without mindfulness you get very little out of your experiences. Life is colourless and unsatisfying. Things happen but you hardly remember them because you never really experienced them in the first place. With mindfulness everything becomes more interesting, more satisfying and more powerful – and more able to crowd out your pain.

Remember this

It isn't necessary to have lots and lots of different things to do. 'Focusing on the present' doesn't require that. On the contrary, you could just sit quietly watching clouds pass by. But make sure that, whatever it is, you're completely focused on it.

Try it now

Think of something that will automatically jog your memory several times a day. It could be passing through a particular doorway, for example, or having a cup of coffee. If nothing springs to mind, simply set your watch or mobile phone to alert you once an hour. Whatever the signal, when you get it, check whether or not you're 'in the present moment'. If you're not, put your thoughts on pause and spend five minutes fully exploring everything around you using all of your senses. Keep on with this technique until mindfulness has become a habit.

COMMITMENT

So that's the 'acceptance' and 'mindfulness' part of ACT. The other major element is 'commitment' to actions that will improve your life, at the same time avoiding actions that are harmful. So it's an essential part of ACT that you should reject harmful pain relief strategies. Psychologists call the use of these harmful strategies 'experiential avoidance'. Some people, for example, eat for comfort, become seriously overweight, and increase their musculoskeletal (MSK) pain as a result. Others rely too much on alcohol which can actually increase anxiety, add the pain of hangover into the equation, and interfere with medication. Yet others turn to recreational drugs and become addicted.

If you conclude that your strategies don't work, or if you conclude they have too high a cost, you may find ACT, or another of the MCA strategies, is the way forward, possibly even the highly controversial TMS approach.

Tension myositis syndrome (TMS)

In 1996, the New York Times published an article entitled 'In One Country, Chronic Whiplash is Uncompensated (and Unknown)'. The country referred to was Lithuania. The article contrasted it with Norway, in which there were '70,000 people in a patients' organization who feel they have chronic disability because of whiplash'. Dr Harald Schrader, a neurologist at University Hospital in Trondheim, Norway, described the situation as 'mass hysteria' given that the population of Norway at the time was only about one-third higher than in Lithuania.

Dr Schrader led a team that went to Lithuania and gave health questionnaires to 202 drivers whose cars had been struck from behind one to three years earlier. They found no one who had 'disabling or persistent symptoms as a result of the car accident'. The conclusion of his study was that whiplash syndrome 'has little validity'.

No doubt some of the Norwegian cases were simple financial opportunism. But in many other instances people genuinely considered themselves to be significantly disabled by whiplash. How could it be?

Dr John Sarno, a retired Professor of Rehabilitation Medicine, believes he knows the answer. He calls it tension myositis syndrome or TMS and he describes it as 'a painful but harmless change of state in muscles'. (Myositis means physiologic alteration of muscles.)

Your doctor may or may not have heard of TMS. You certainly won't find it in standard medical textbooks. TMS is, in fact, the discovery – some would say, invention – of Dr Sarno. He claims it's 'the most common emotionally induced disorder in the United States, and probably in the Western world'. It is his contention that certain cases of physical pain are caused by the brain or, more specifically, the unconscious mind.

Why would the brain do that? Most people, including doctors, nowadays would accept that there is a mind body connection. But Dr Sarno's theory takes it to a whole new level. It is his contention that the brain can create pain, and certain other distressing conditions, as a distraction. He sees it as akin to a conjuror distracting an audience or to a criminal setting a fire in one place so a robbery can be committed in another.

Right now you may be saying 'ridiculous' or you may be nodding your head in recognition. What is beyond dispute is that the 'bodymind' can injure itself. We know for a fact that there are, for example, autoimmune diseases in which the immune system mistakes some part of the body as a pathogen and attacks it. Examples include coeliac disease, Crohn's disease, Diabetes mellitus type 1, Lupus erythematosus, psoriasis, and rheumatoid arthritis.

So far, so logical.

Where Dr Sarno's ideas get most controversial is in his explanation for why the bodymind deliberately creates pain. For what reason would your unconscious deliberately damage the body in which it resides? What awful thing could justify such a terrible diversion?

According to Dr Sarno, it's all down to what he calls 'narcissistic rage'. Narcissistic rage is the uncontrollable anger that results from a narcissistic injury – a threat to a person's self-esteem or worth.

According to Dr Sarno we all have six basic needs. They are:

▶ To be perfect (to excel, to succeed)

▶ To be liked

▶ To be taken care of

▶ To be soothed (through food, drink, sex, entertainment and so on)

▶ To be physically invincible

▶ To be immortal.

As Dr Sarno sees it, these needs are almost impossible to fulfil. No one is perfect. Some people are widely liked but no one is universally liked and most of us have only a few close friends.

Unless we're unlucky, we have at least one person who will take care of us to a degree, but we may find that it's we who are expected to look after others. We certainly can be soothed by food, drink, music, sex and so on, and yet it's never quite enough. As for invincibility and immortality, we're all too soon confronted with the horrible reality that we get old, ill and die.

Because our needs can't be met we're in this constant state of narcissistic rage. You may deny it, but you wouldn't be consciously aware of it because it would be repressed in your unconscious mind. And it's in order to keep it repressed that the unconscious creates diversionary pains and illnesses.

Let's leave Dr Sarno's explanation of the unconscious motive aside. You may find it very hard to accept. But it's not essential to Dr Sarno's case. We know for a fact that there are psychogenic disorders (caused, intensified or prolonged by emotional, mental or behavioural factors). Could back pain, Dr Sarno's speciality, be one of them?

Key idea

Although a history of sexual abuse increases the chances of suffering various chronic illnesses later in life, having one of those illnesses is not confirmation that you were abused. In a French study, one third of IBS sufferers had been abused but the majority had not been.

TMS AND BACK PAIN

Dr Sarno is sceptical of the notion that after millions of years of evolution the human back is incapable of taking a little strain or unable to carry out repairs. He cites various studies in which large numbers of people with protruding discs and other abnormalities nevertheless did not suffer back pain. Why not?

When Dr Sarno analysed his own patients' case notes he found that 88 per cent had 'a history of minor gastrointestinal maladies such as heartburn, pre-ulcer symptoms, hiatus hernia, colitis, spastic colon, irritable bowel syndrome and other tension-induced reactions like tension headache, migraine headache, eczema and frequent urination.' Dr Sarno believes that what separates many people with chronic pain from those without are psychological or emotional phenomena.

DO DR SARNO'S METHODS WORK?

In 1982 Dr Sarno made his first survey. One hundred and seventy-seven patients with back pain were selected at random from those who had been treated by him between 1978 and 1981. Seventy-six per cent were said to be leading normal lives and were 'essentially pain free', 8 per cent were 'somewhat improved' and 16 per cent were considered 'treatment failures'.

Dr Sarno improved his methods and when a second survey was carried out in 1987 his success rate was even higher. One to three years after treatment by the 'Sarno method':

▶ 88 per cent were free of pain and leading normal lives

▶ 10 per cent were 'somewhat better'

▶ 2 per cent were unchanged.

It should be remembered that these were all people with back pain that was chronic. What's more, those in the second survey were men and women with CT-scanned documented herniated discs – the abnormality that's responsible for most back surgery in the USA.

It has to be said that these figures are Dr Sarno's own. We have no independent, double-blind trials. But we do have corroboration of sorts from satisfied patients, including some high profile celebrities.

THE SARNO METHOD

Dr Sarno certainly agrees with those who say back pain is caused by a reduction in oxygen to the tissues involved. He also agrees that the oxygen deprivation is often due to physical blockages in the arteries. Where he departs from mainstream medicine is in his insistence that the unconscious mind can inhibit the blood supply to particular tissues.

You won't be able to consult Dr Sarno personally. Born in 1923, he retired long ago. Nor will you easily find doctors following his methods (but you'll find some at www.tmswiki.org).

So can you apply Dr Sarno's methods to yourself? Up to a certain extent, you can. But before you can even start you have to believe that your back pain (or whatever it is) could have originated in your brain. Dr Sarno's experience is that people who reject a psychological explanation do not respond to his method. So if you're already saying 'Rubbish! Rubbish!' this isn't going to work for you.

Here, then, is the Sarno method:

1 Make a list of all the things you're angry about from your childhood.

2 Make a list of all the pressures you're subject to now (including pressures associated with nice things).

3 Spend time every day meditating on the things in your present and past life that put you under pressure and cause rage.

4 Frequently repeat something like this: 'I have a normal back (or whatever). I now know that my condition was initiated by my brain to serve a psychological purpose.' In the case of back pain you might also add: 'The physical abnormalities that have been found are simply normal changes associated with activity and ageing.'

5 Whenever you have pain, deliberately think about your repressed rage and the reasons for it. This, as it were, undoes the strategy of the unconscious mind, which is to stop you thinking about your repressed rage.

6 Tell your unconscious you know what it's up to. Say you know the pain is harmless and that it's a technique of distraction. In the case of backache, order your unconscious to increase the blood flow.

7 Once the pain is diminishing, begin the resumption of normal physical activities.

If this doesn't work for you, it may be that the cause of your problems is so well repressed that you just can't uncover it without professional help. If that's what you suspect then you should consider psychotherapy to get at the truth about your past.

OBJECTIONS TO TMS

One day in 1984, Barry Marshall picked up a dish containing the bacterium *Helicobacter pylori* and drank it. He didn't know for sure what would happen but he had a good idea. He and his colleague Robert Warren had theorized that bacteria, and not stress, were responsible for stomach ulcers. It was a theory that had been widely derided and there seemed to be only one way to know for sure.

Three days later Marshall developed nausea and bad breath. Five days later he began vomiting. Eight days later an endoscopy revealed massive inflammation – the bacteria were everywhere in his stomach. Ten days later his wife told him she'd had enough of his experiment. He took antibiotics, the bacteria were killed, and the inflammation went away. So, for many, did the idea that ulcers had a psychological cause. And that cast doubt on the psychological explanation for many other conditions.

It seemed an open and shut case. Bacteria, not stress, caused ulcers. But Dr Sarno was not put off. He points out that *H. pylori* has probably occupied the guts of humans and their predecessors for millions of years. What's more, as many as a third of all adults in the West seem to carry it, rising to half by age 65. But only about a fifth go on to develop gastric diseases like ulcers. Why? Dr Sarno remains convinced that the difference between those who suffer ulcers and those who get along with their *H. Pylori* is down to emotional factors.

A more obvious objection to the theory of TMS is this. Most people would probably say they'd happily face up to the contents of their unconscious minds if that meant the end of physical pain. Dr Sarno's answer is that the unconscious is not very rational. It acts, he says, like a child in a tantrum.

Personally, I'm not sure that I buy this view. The unconscious mind is awesomely powerful and wonderfully analytical. How could it be so wrong? However, it's not necessary to accept that particular explanation in order to accept TMS. The basic premise works without narcissistic rage and without defence mechanisms. Just hold onto the main idea which is that the brain, for whatever reason, can be the originator of the pain. When it is, the treatment must be psychological.

Focus points

* CBT teaches that the cognitions (thoughts) you have about your pain can make it better or worse.
* ACT teaches that it's possible to detach from pain and therefore feel it less keenly.
* Mindfulness teaches that by focusing on the present moment you can crowd out pain.
* According to the theory of TMS, pain may be due to a reduction in blood flow caused by the unconscious mind.
* The TMS solution is to deal with past mental traumas and present stress, thus restoring blood flow and curing the pain.

Next step

In this chapter and the previous one we've covered the mental approach to pain fairly comprehensively. In the next chapter we're going to be looking at something much more tangible. We'll be seeing how eating the wrong things can cause pain and how eating the right things can cure it. And there's nothing 'wacky' about it. There's plenty of scientific evidence to prove it.

Foods that fight pain

In this chapter you will learn:

▶ *how food can cause pain*
▶ *how food can cure pain*
▶ *how to develop an 'anti-pain' diet.*

One should eat nutritious food and exercise regularly to have sound health

The Rig Veda, one of the oldest written books
(1700–1100 BCE)

How could what you eat have any bearing on the pain you feel in your knees? Or in your head? Or your back? It hardly seems possible. And yet it's true. Food has been described as both the cause of the majority of human ailments and as a pharmacy. What you eat has a very real bearing on the illnesses you suffer, the diseases you avoid, and the pain you feel.

For example, food can:

▶ Reduce inflammation

▶ Reduce the brain's sensitivity to pain

▶ Have an analgesic effect on nerves

▶ Protect the digestive tract.

On the other hand, food can also:

▶ Cause inflammation (leading to painful joints)

▶ Cause allergies (which are sometimes painful)

▶ Cause arterial plaque (which can block arteries leading to pain and even heart attack)

▶ Cause kidney stones (which are always painful).

So you may be able to cure pain by consuming certain foods. Equally, you may be able to prevent pain by avoiding certain foods.

Why should it be that some foods are 'dangerous'. One theory is that we can't cope with 'unnatural' foods, that's to say, foods unavailable to our pre-Stone Age ancestors. And, in fact, the most common food suspects in the case of migraine, arthritis, fibromyalgia, irritable bowel syndrome and Crohn's disease are all things that have been introduced into the human diet relatively recently. They are:

▶ Meat

▶ Dairy products

- Chickens' eggs
- Wheat
- Corn
- Certain nuts
- Tomatoes
- Citrus Fruits
- Caffeine.

It is only a theory. But, whatever the reason, the impact of food on health and pain is beyond dispute. Let's now take a look at your diet.

Diagnostic test

1 My diet is (a) low in fat (b) average in fat (c) high in fat.

2 I am (a) a vegan (b) a vegetarian (c) a person who can't go without meat.

3 I eat plenty of (a) fruit and vegetables (b) meat and fish.

4 I (a) never add salt to food (b) use salt very carefully (c) love salty things.

5 I (a) eat plenty of green leafy vegetables and legumes (b) hate cabbage, sprouts, broccoli and all that stuff.

6 I (a) eat plenty of whole grains (b) prefer white bread, white rice and ordinary pasta.

7 I (a) eat garlic every day (b) eat garlic at least once a week (c) never eat garlic.

8 I have had my blood tested and my cholesterol is (a) under 150 mg/dl (3.9 mmol/l) (b) between 150 mg/dl (3.9 mmol/l) and 240 mg/dl (6.2 mmol/l) (c) over 240 mg/dl (6.2 mmol/l).

9 I (a) almost never get migraines or headaches (b) often get migraines or headaches.

10 I (a) eat for health (b) eat for taste (c) eat for comfort.

Foods that reduce inflammation

As we saw in Chapter 1, special cells in your body can cause inflammation. They're a good thing if you're under attack by some kind of infection or have suffered an injury. Their aim is to:

▶ Increase the flow of blood (thus causing the redness and heat)

▶ Allow white cells from the blood into the tissues to fight disease-causing organisms (thus causing the swelling)

▶ Immobilize the area (thus causing stiffness)

▶ Protect the area from further damage (by sending pain signals).

Normally, as soon as the problem has been dealt with the inflammation subsides and the pain goes. But there are a number of diseases including acne, asthma, coeliac disease, chronic prostatitis, inflammatory bowel disease and rheumatoid arthritis, in which inflammation goes wild.

One of the chemicals that causes inflammation is known as prostaglandin E_2 and it's made in the body from certain fatty acids in the food you eat. The main culprits are:

▶ Arachidonic acid in meat, dairy products and eggs

▶ Linoleic acid in certain vegetable oils, especially safflower oil, grape seed oil, sunflower oil, corn oil, cottonseed oil and soybean oil.

These fats become incorporated into the membranes of your cells. Most healthy people tolerate normal quantities of dietary arachidonic and linoleic acids perfectly well, but some do not. In their case, prostaglandin E_2 gets released when it's not needed. Changing the nature of your cell membranes won't stop you releasing prostaglandin E_2 altogether (nor would you want that) but it will help prevent it being released inappropriately.

If you suffer pain from an inflammatory disease such as rheumatoid arthritis your path is clear. You need to eliminate arachidonic and linoleic acids from your diet and see what happens. Other 'trigger' foods for some people are:

- Corn
- Citrus fruits
- Potatoes
- Tomatoes
- Nuts
- Coffee.

Try it now

Starting today, completely cut out the sources of arachidonic and linoleic acid and the other 'trigger foods' mentioned above and make the following the mainstay of your diet for one month, since they're seldom involved in inflammatory reactions:

- Brown rice
- Cooked green, yellow and orange vegetables
- Cooked or dried cherries, cranberries, pears or prunes
- Water
- Salt, maple syrup and vanilla as flavourings.

In place of your usual vegetable oils substitute:

- Flaxseed/linseed oil (high in alpha-linolenic acid or ALA)
- Starflower oil/borage oil (high in gamma-linolenic acid or GLA).

You can eat and drink other things, as long as they're not on the 'trigger' list, but only in small amounts. If your symptoms have improved by the end of the month you'll know that something in your old way of eating was at least partly to blame. You can then reintroduce foods, at the rate of one every two days. In particular, reintroduce the following, which have anti-inflammatory properties:

- Blackberries
- Blueberries
- Cayenne pepper
- Celery and celery seeds
- Fish/fish oil
- Ginger
- Raspberries
- Strawberries
- Turmeric
- Walnuts.

If your symptoms worsen after consuming a certain food or drink then you have your culprit.

Remember this

It's a pretty tough regime but it's only for a while. Once you've identified the problem food or foods you can return to eating everything else. Don't give up after a couple of weeks because you see no improvement. It usually takes about four weeks to notice any effect from changing your diet, and it can take several months to optimally convert your cell walls. Be patient and give the process time to work.

Foods that clean arteries

How could fast food give you backache? At first sight it doesn't seem credible. And yet it's perfectly logical. It could also increase your chances of, among other serious and painful dramas, heart attack, stroke and peripheral artery disease (PAD), which makes it difficult to run or walk without discomfort. What all these things have in common is reduced blood supply due to blockages in the blood vessels.

Blockages contain cholesterol (a fatty substance known as a lipid) which is why the American Heart Association, along with many other respected bodies, is quite clear that a type known as LDL cholesterol is a risk factor. They argue that dietary cholesterol needs to be reduced. In other words, much less fast food and much less fat (especially animal fat) in the diet.

If you haven't done so recently your first step should be to visit your doctor and have your cholesterol level checked. Here, according to mainstream medical opinion, is how to interpret the results.

Cholesterol	Health risk
Under 3.9 mmol/l (under 150 mg/dl)	Very low
3.9 – 5.2 mmol/l (150 – 200 mg/dl)	Low to average
5.2 – 6.2 mmol/l (200 – 240 mg/dl)	Above average
Over 6.2 mmol/l (over 240 mg/dl)	Very high

I say 'according to mainstream medical opinion' because cholesterol is controversial in two ways. Firstly, some scientists dispute that cholesterol is the cause of the problem. Secondly, even if it is, a significant body of opinion doubts that it can be controlled by diet. That's because we all manufacture far more cholesterol than we eat. And we do that because it's essential for life and is a major component of cell walls.

To put things into perspective, a man of 68 kg (150 pounds) will have around 35 g of cholesterol in his body and will make around 1 g a day. Against that, meat-eating adult Westerners typically consume 300 – 600 mg of cholesterol every day, which would account for up to 0.6 mmol/l in their blood cholesterol reading. That's only about ten per cent of the average person's cholesterol.

Many doctors therefore doubt that reducing the cholesterol in the diet can achieve very much (and not all of it is absorbed, anyway). Their response would be to control cholesterol through medication.

But the emphasis on the intake of cholesterol misses something very important. Incredible as it may seem:

▶ There are foods that actually reduce the body's production of cholesterol.

These foods, then, go right to the root of the problem. The more of them you eat, the lower your cholesterol will go.

The most important of these cholesterol-reducing foods are:

▶ Barley. Barley contains an abundance of tocotrienol, a member of the vitamin E family, which suppresses the liver's ability to produce cholesterol. In a 1993 study at the Kenneth Jordan Heart Foundation and Elmhurst Medical Center, seven of nine high cholesterol patients taking tocotrienols actually experienced reversal of the narrowing of their arteries. The other two worsened, but, by comparison, in a control group not taking tocotrienols, none improved and ten worsened. So that's extremely positive for barley.

▶ Oats. Oat bran has been found to be effective in about 85 per cent of people. In 1997 the Food and Drug Administration (FDA) of the USA approved a health claim that a substance called β-glucan in oats reduced plasma cholesterol levels. A 2011 study at the University of Manitoba, Canada, found that 3 g of oat β-glucan a day could reduce LDL cholesterol by between 5 and 10 per cent.

▶ Wheat and rye. These two also contain tocotrienol, but in smaller quantities than barley does.

▶ Walnuts. A study published in the American Journal for Clinical Nutrition in 2001 concluded that, when added to the normal diet, a handful of walnuts daily could lower LDL levels by 27 per cent.

▶ Other 'anti-cholesterol' foods include dried beans, and the flesh and membranes of grapefruit.

There are also certain nutritional deficiencies and certain foods that are believed to increase the risk of atherosclerosis (plaque in the arteries). They include:

▶ Vitamin B6 deficiency. This is uncommon but the elderly, alcoholics, those with HIV and those on certain medicaments are vulnerable. Good sources of B6 include meat, whole grains, vegetables, nuts and bananas.

▶ Iodine deficiency. A 1933 study found that iodine protected rabbits on a high-cholesterol diet from atherosclerosis. According to one source, 16.5 per cent of Americans were deficient in iodine in 2005, partly due to a reduced intake of iodized salt. Good sources of iodine include sea vegetables, yoghurt, milk, eggs and strawberries.

▶ Trans fats. Trans fats in the diet come mostly from the processed food industry as a result of the hydrogenation of unsaturated plant fats. You can avoid them by cutting out fast foods, commercial fried foods and commercial baked goods. Some food companies are making an effort to reduce or eliminate trans fats in their products – check food labels carefully.

▶ Rancid fats. When fat is exposed to air it oxidizes – that's to say, it becomes rancid. The higher the temperature, the quicker it happens. Rancid fat doesn't taste very pleasant and most people would automatically reject it. But a little oxidation will probably go unnoticed. Buy vegetable oils in small bottles so you can use them quickly and store them in the fridge. If there's no room in the fridge, at least keep them in a cool, dark place with the lids on.

▶ Obesity. Obesity does not directly increase the risk of atherosclerosis but it may do so indirectly by increasing the risk of high blood pressure. In turn, high blood pressure can damage the walls of the arteries, creating the conditions for the deposition of the plaque that causes blockages.

Try it now

Use barley in your very next meal. You can substitute it for rice, for example, in a risotto. Or you could use barley flour, together with oats, to make biscuits. For a full range of barley recipes see allrecipes.co.uk.

Food and kidney pain

Kidney stones cause severe pain in the back and especially when urinating. Those who have suffered them often describe the pain as the worst they have ever experienced. But kidney stones can be avoided very simply by modifying what you eat. Most are composed of calcium oxalate, a combination of the calcium and oxalate in the typical diet. A minority of stones are composed of uric acid, formed by the breakdown of protein.

You can minimize your risk by:

- Drinking about 2.5 litres of liquid a day
- Not adding salt to food
- Eating high potassium/low salt foods such as fresh bananas, black beans, haricot beans and cauliflower
- Reducing your consumption of meat, dairy and eggs
- Eliminating sugar.

Food, cancer and cancer pain

Anthony J Sattilaro was a doctor in Philadelphia who, in 1978, was diagnosed with prostate cancer that had spread to his skull, his spine and a rib. The rib and both of his testicles were removed (in accordance with the belief that testosterone fuels prostate cancer). It was hoped that would provide a remission but six weeks later things were still bleak and the doctors prescribed the 'female' hormone oestrogen. He was on morphine and cocaine for pain as well as compazine to control vomiting.

Then, according to his book *Recalled by Life*, Sattilaro experienced a second life-changing event. He picked up two hitch-hikers. Chatting as he drove along he revealed that he had little time to live. One of the hitchhikers told him: 'You don't have to die; cancer isn't all that hard to cure.' The solution, they said, was a macrobiotic diet, such as they followed. Dr Sattilaro reasoned he had nothing to lose. He consulted Denny Waxman, director of the Philadelphia East West Foundation. The basic macrobiotic diet is 50 per cent cooked whole grains, 25 per cent locally grown vegetables, 15 per cent beans and sea vegetables and 10 per cent fruits, nuts, seeds and fish. In view of Dr Sattilaro's dangerous condition, Waxman recommended an even more restricted diet initially without fish, oil, flour products or fruit.

Two weeks later, according to Dr Sattilaro's own account, the majority of the pain had disappeared. At that point he was still on the oestrogen therapy but by June 1979 he stopped it. He continued to feel better and in September, 15 months after starting macrobiotics, new scans were unable to detect any cancer in his skull or spine.

What was due to conventional cancer treatment, what was due to nutrition, and what was due to some other unidentified factor, is impossible to know. But it's now believed that the wrong food contributes to between 30 and 60 per cent of cancers.

In 1986 Dr Sattilaro was interviewed by Dr Neal Barnard and told him that he intended to reintroduce animal protein into his diet. Barnard cautioned against it but Sattilaro was a little bored with his restricted diet and also curious to know what would happen. What did happen is that his cancer returned and he died in 1989.

Of course, it can't be proved that once again eating animal protein was the cause of the relapse. It could have been coincidence. But prostate cancer is consistently linked with animal products, especially those that are high in fats. The same is true for breast cancer. In one study in Buffalo, New York, researchers concluded that for women with breast cancer that had spread, their risk of dying at any given moment increased 40 per cent for every thousand grams of fat consumed per month. The same is also believed to be the case for cancer of the uterus and ovary. To put that in perspective, the average Western woman consumes around 2,000 grams of fat per month. Switching to a well-planned vegan diet could cut that to 600 grams.

Indeed, there are many stories like Dr Sattilaro's. Always the problem is in proving that the diet made a difference over and above the conventional treatment. So what should you do? Look at it this way. If you're suffering from cancer pain then, like Dr Sattilaro, you have nothing to lose by following an 'anti-cancer diet', except a little of the pleasure that comes with food.

But isn't it worth a go?

Try it now

Try a vegan or macrobiotic diet for a month and see if it helps reduce your pain. It will come as less of a shock if you make sure you're never hungry (which is certain to cause a craving for the foods you're used to). Get a good recipe book, think it through carefully, and make sure you have all the meat, cheese, egg and milk substitutes in your cupboard before you begin.

Food allergies and food intolerance

Allergies and food intolerance are on the increase. In fact, allergic diseases are the most common cause of chronic illness in developed countries. We don't know why, but industrialization and urban living somehow seem to have something to do with it. A survey of 30 countries carried out for the World Allergy Organization (WAO) found allergy rates of 40 per cent in Japan and the Ukraine, but only 7.5 per cent in Colombia. In another study, the allergy rate for 13 – 14 year olds in Greece was found to be 3.7 per cent but in the UK 32.2 per cent. In a third study of more than 4,500 adults from 13 Western countries, the rate of food sensitivity (as measured by antibodies in the blood) ranged from 8% in Reykjavik in Iceland to 25% in Portland, Oregon. Interestingly, the foods that caused the allergies tended to be the same everywhere:

▶ Hazelnuts, peaches, shrimps, wheat and apples turned out to be the most common culprits globally

▶ Cow's milk, eggs, soya, peanuts, other nuts, fish and shellfish are other common allergens.

Allergies are caused by the immune system producing antibodies known as class E immunoglobulins (IgE), which are the body's normal response to parasitic infections. We don't know why there should be an inappropriate and exaggerated response to other substances. Another mystery is that a third of people who produce excess IgE nevertheless show no other signs of an allergic reaction.

Symptoms of allergy may include:

▶ Headache/migraine

▶ Heartburn

▶ Joint stiffness

▶ Colitis (inflammation of the large intestine)

▶ Cystitis (inflammation of the bladder)

▶ Runny nose and streaming eyes

▶ Conjunctivitis (irritation of the eyes)

▶ Skin rashes

▶ Swelling of the lips and tongue

- Breathing difficulties
- Abdominal swelling
- Fatigue.

Although an allergy sounds worse than an intolerance, the possible symptoms of intolerance are actually more wide-ranging. They include:

- Headaches
- Joint pain
- Muscle pain
- Stomach ache
- Bloating
- Irritable bowel syndrome (IBS)
- Gastroesophageal Reflux Disease (GERD)
- Asthma
- Eczema
- Skin rashes
- Depression, irritability, anxiety and panic attacks
- Fatigue, forgetfulness and brain fog.

Key idea

There are several important differences between food allergy and food intolerance:

* Food allergy is an immune reaction whereas intolerance is the result of an enzyme deficiency or excess. The standard IgE antibody tests will therefore show if you're allergic to certain things but they won't show whether or not you have an intolerance.

* An allergic reaction usually occurs within seconds or minutes whereas the symptoms of a food intolerance usually appear within minutes, hours or even days.

* Allergies are limited to one genus of foods whereas intolerance is not limited to genus but to chemicals that may be common to many foods.

* Allergies do not affect the nervous system but food intolerance can.

Remember this

Nowadays, the standard response to allergy and food intolerance is to take antihistamines. They work very well and, sometimes, there is no alternative. But antihistamines can have side effects, including sleepiness, foggy brain, dry mouth, dizziness, a tight feeling in the chest, rapid heart beat and erection difficulties. So it makes sense to try to track down the source of the problem as described below.

TACKLING ALLERGY AND FOOD INTOLERANCE

Occasionally the cause of a symptom can be very plain. If you'd never had a reaction before in your life until, say, 15 minutes after taking a new medicament, the trigger would be fairly obvious. But things are rarely that simple. Some reactions are as quick as that but others can take far longer, making it very difficult to identify the culprit.

The only DIY method of identifying an allergen or a problem food is to restrict your diet and at the same time keep a meticulous food, drink and allergy diary. This is known as the 'elimination test'.

Here's what to do:

1 Reduce the variety of things you eat and drink to no more than ten – fewer would be better. Focus on things that are the least likely to be the cause of your symptoms. Rice makes an excellent foundation for an elimination diet because it rarely causes a problem and is extremely versatile. It can be sweet or savoury and you can even drink it as rice milk. Don't use any herbs or spices with it – or with anything else. (But see the warning about rice below.)

2 Whenever you swallow anything make sure you record: the time; the source of the food or drink (canned peas, for example, might cause a response but frozen peas might not); whether or not it was cooked (a particular fruit, for example, might cause an allergic response when raw but not when cooked).

3 Continue until your symptoms have cleared up (maximum four weeks). Then reintroduce foods at the rate of one every three days. On the first day use just a little, on the second

day more, and on the third day a normal portion. If you get no response you can assume the food is probably safe and incorporate it into your normal diet. If you do get a response then you have your culprit.

4 If there's no improvement at the end of four weeks then it may be the culprit is one of the few things you're still eating or drinking. Or it may be you'll have to consider a different approach.

▶ Warning

Do not follow the reintroduction procedure if you've experienced a severe allergic reaction in the past. Reintroducing an allergen might trigger anaphylactic shock, which could be fatal if not treated immediately.

▶ Warning

In the last few years concern has been mounting over the arsenic content of rice. A study released by Consumer Reports in 2012 found levels typically from three to seven micrograms per serving and in some cases even higher. By way of a yardstick, the federal limit for drinking water in the USA is 10 parts per billion, which equates to 10 micrograms per litre. In other words, eating a meal in which rice formed a substantial part could be roughly equal to drinking a litre of water at the federal limit for arsenic contamination. Organic Indian Basmati and Organic Thai Jasmine appear to be among the safest types. Experts recommend thoroughly washing the rice and cooking it in an excess of water to reduce the arsenic content.

HISTAMINE AND SALICYLATES

There's always the possibility that it takes two, three or even more foods acting together to cause a response. When you eat one, nothing happens. When you eat three you get a reaction.

If you suspect that's what's happening, you could be intolerant of histamine or salicylates, chemicals naturally occurring in a wide variety of foods.

Histamine is a very clever substance. It's a neurotransmitter, it regulates the functioning of the gut, and it increases the permeability of the capillaries to allow white blood cells out into the surrounding tissues to fight pathogens, which is part of the inflammatory response. Some foods and drinks contain histamine and they normally cause no problem. But if you're deficient in the enzyme diamine oxidase you may get allergy-like symptoms such as headache, stomach pains and rashes.

High levels of histamine occur in:

▶ Red wine and champagne

▶ Pickled foods

▶ Foods containing vinegar

▶ Tofu and soya sauce

▶ Cheese

▶ Processed meats

▶ Mushrooms

▶ Quorn

▶ Dried fruit, seeds and nuts

▶ Yeast and yeast extract

▶ Chocolate and cocoa

▶ Cola

▶ Prepared salads and tinned vegetables.

There are also foods that, while containing little histamine, nevertheless stimulate histamine production in the body. They include:

▶ Spices

▶ Tomatoes

▶ Shellfish

▶ Spinach

▶ Egg white

▶ Many fruits.

If you notice that you have a problem when you, say, eat a tomato and mushroom sauce with parmesan cheese, washed down with red wine, but that you can eat any of those things individually, then histamine intolerance should be suspected. In that case, avoid food and drink in the two lists above and see what happens.

Salicylates are derivatives of salicylic acid, which plants use to protect themselves from bacteria, fungi and insects. In other words, when you eat plant foods you're eating the poisons that plants use to defend themselves. Humans normally cope perfectly well with them and, indeed, willow bark, with its high level of salicin was long used to treat headaches and fever. But some people are intolerant of salicylates and that might include you if you suffer from:

▶ Unexplained headaches

▶ Stomach pain

▶ Fatigue

▶ Nausea

▶ Breathing difficulties

▶ Rashes

▶ Swelling of the hands, feet, lips and skin around the eyes

▶ Urgent need to urinate.

Unfortunately, salicylates are impossible to avoid entirely, but you can try to reduce your consumption. Foods that contain high levels of salicylates include:

▶ Most fruits (except bananas, golden delicious apples, limes, papayas and pears)

▶ Most vegetables (except beans, cabbage, celery, lettuce, swede and white potatoes)

▶ Most nuts and seeds (except cashews, hazelnuts, pecans, poppy seeds and sunflower seeds)

▶ Most fats and oils (except butter, canola/rapeseed, safflower, soya and sunflower)

- ▶ Corn/maize
- ▶ Seasoned meats
- ▶ Coffee, tea and fruit juices
- ▶ Alcoholic drinks (except gin, whisky and vodka).

If you suspect salicylate intolerance, avoid high-salicylate food and drink for a while and see what happens. You can find a full list of salicylate-containing foods at: http://salicylatesensitivity.com/

Key idea

Fruits and vegetables have their highest salicylate content when they're unripe so always wait until they're a little over-ripe before eating them.

Try it now

There is no laboratory test for salicylate intolerance. If you suspect it see your doctor at once and ask him or her to supervise a 'provocative challenge' by giving higher and higher doses of aspirin, until intolerance either appears or is ruled out.

Food and migraine

Migraine is a horribly disabling condition. In addition to a throbbing pain in the head, usually on just one side, symptoms may include sensitivity to light and noise, nausea, vomiting, disturbances to vision, lack of co-ordination and, in extreme cases, partial paralysis. Even after the attack is over, sufferers may experience a 'hangover' lasting several hours before they feel normal again.

Incredibly, food and drink can be migraine triggers, either acting alone or in combination with other factors. Here are the worst culprits:

- ▶ Dairy products
- ▶ Chocolate
- ▶ Eggs

- Citrus fruits
- Preserved meat and fish
- Wheat
- Nuts
- Tomatoes
- Onions
- Corn
- Apples
- Bananas
- Alcohol, especially red wine
- Coffee, tea, colas and other caffeinated beverages
- Monosodium glutamate
- Aspartame (artificial sweetener)
- Missing a meal
- Missing your usual quantity of caffeinated drinks (caffeine withdrawal).

Foods that are very unlikely to cause migraine include:

- Brown rice
- Dried or cooked fruits (but apples, bananas, citrus fruits, peaches and tomatoes might be culprits)
- Cooked vegetables (except root vegetables and green leafy vegetables)
- Water (including carbonated water).

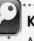

Key idea

A migraine could be triggered by something you ate or drank as much as 48 hours ago. The best way of discovering your problem foods is to keep a diary. It will be a bit of a chore because it needs to be very meticulous. But if it stops your attacks it will be well worth the effort. It should include:

* Everything you eat and drink and at what time
* What time you go to bed and get up
* Everything you do (work, exercise, watch TV etc.)
* When you go to the toilet
* Your mood
* The weather
* Menstrual cycle
* Migraine attacks.

Detail is essential because it may be that you only get an attack when several factors are combined.

Remember this

Nitrites can cause migraines. They're used to preserve fish and meat but they're also formed when nitrates in root vegetables and green leafy vegetables (especially lettuce and spinach) are converted into nitrites in the body. A high intake of vitamin C helps prevent nitrites forming.

Case study

'For about three years I had migraine attacks that began as a pain behind one eye. Curiously, they mostly struck in the winter but only rarely in the summer. Many winter mornings I would awaken with this eye pain even though I had felt fine when I went to bed. Gradually it would extend into a full headache and I would feel kind of unco-ordinated. I suspected glaucoma, but my pressure was fine, and my eye specialist could find nothing wrong. Then I suspected the gloomy winter light was causing eyestrain but even on sunny winter days I still had the problem. Next I blamed the long artificially lit nights. But as the days lengthened the number of attacks stayed the same. Then I thought it might be the temperature in the bedroom but turning up the central heating made no difference. I was in despair because I could be wiped out for an entire day. Finally I realized there was one other difference between summer and

Foods, herbs and supplements that reduce pain

In the following section you'll find a wide variety of foods,
herbs and supplements that act as medicaments for pain. Many
of them can be incorporated into your regular diet, others
will have to be taken as pills. Don't underestimate the power
of plants. They were the origin of some of our most powerful
pharmaceuticals.

ALPHA-LIPOIC ACID

▶ **What will it do for me?**

Alpha-lipoic acid reduces neuropathic pain for some sufferers,
especially when the pain is a side effect of diabetes. It also seems
to help for a number of other conditions by preventing certain
kinds of cell damage. Some sufferers find it reduces migraine
attacks. It's an antioxidant and found in low levels in broccoli,
peas, potatoes, spinach, yeast and some offal, as well as being
made in the body.

▶ **How should I use it?**

As a supplement, the standard dose for treating type 2 diabetes
and relieving pain, burning and numbness is 600 – 1200 mg.

▶ **Any side effects?**

Not many. Some people get a rash. If you're a heavy drinker
or know you have a thiamine deficiency you should take a
thiamine supplement. Alpha-lipoic acid may interfere with
treatments for an underactive or overactive thyroid gland. If
you have diabetes you may need to adjust your medication
as alpha-lipoic acid can reduce blood sugar. As a precaution,
alpha-lipoic acid supplements should not be taken by women
who are pregnant or breastfeeding.

BOSWELLIA SERRATA

▶ What will it do for me?

Resin from Boswellia serrata (also known as Indian frankincense) has long been used in Ayurvedic medicine as an anti-inflammatory. Western science has now proven that, among other effects, it blocks the pro-inflammatory enzyme 5-LOX. In one study, 82 per cent of those who took Boswellia experienced complete remission from ulcerative colitis. In another study conducted at the Barmherzige Schwestern Hospital in Linz, Austria, Boswellia was found to be effective in reducing the intensity and frequency of attacks in those suffering from chronic cluster headaches (CCH). Boswellia appears to have the ability to stabilize mast cells and limit the release of histamine, making it useful for allergy sufferers. As a treatment for osteoarthritis, rheumatoid arthritis and backache, Boswellia generally reduces pain but seems to have little impact on the progress of the conditions themselves.

▶ How should I use it?

The effective dose in most cases is around 300 mg three times daily (at a strength of 60 – 65 per cent boswellic acid). It's also available as a cream for external use on joints.

▶ Any side effects?

Long-term Boswellia use does not seem to lead to irritation or ulceration of the stomach, as can occur with steroids and non-steroidal anti-inflammatory drugs (NSAIDs). However, it's recommended you should take it only for two to three months. Very rarely, side effects include diarrhoea, nausea and skin rash.

BROMELAIN

▶ What will it do for me?

Bromelain is a natural anti-inflammatory and blood thinner derived from the pineapple plant. It has been used in Central and South America for centuries and has been officially approved in Germany for the treatment of swelling following surgery, especially sinus surgery. In one study, three-quarters of surgery patients did better on bromelain than on NSAIDs.

How should I use it?

The German Commission E (Germany's equivalent of the USA's Food and Drug Administration) recommends between 80 mg and 320 mg two to three times a day. As an aid to digestion bromelain should be taken with meals, but for pain caused by injury or arthritis take between meals. It's generally recommended not to take bromelain more than ten days in a row.

Any side effects?

Common side effects include indigestion, nausea and diarrhoea. Less common side effects include drowsiness, vomiting and heavy periods. Some people have allergic reactions – don't take bromelain if you're allergic to pineapples, carrots, celery, fennel, rye, wheat, papain, bee stings, latex, or the pollen from grass, birch or cypress. Don't take if you have peptic ulcers or if you're taking blood thinning medicines/herbs, ACE inhibitors, other drugs that cause drowsiness or are receiving chemotherapy. If you're on antibiotics take medical advice because bromelain increases the absorption of certain kinds.

CAPSAICIN

What will it do for me?

Capsaicin is the chemical that makes chillies hot. A cream containing capsaicin rubbed into the skin will reduce the pain of osteoarthritis and rheumatoid arthritis as well as from damage to nerves near the skin surface (as with shingles, for example). Patients at the New England Centre for Headache reduced the pain of migraine and cluster headaches by applying a little capsaicin cream inside their nostrils. Used externally, capsaicin works by locally depleting a chemical called substance P which transmits pain signals. The effect builds day by day, reaching its maximum after about four weeks, as more and more substance P gets used up. Internally, eating chilli peppers causes the well-known burning sensation, stimulating the body to release endorphins. As a result, there's a general reduction in pain and a mild euphoria. As cayenne pepper, capsaicin may ease the pain of bloating.

▶ How should I use it?

Try a cream of between 0.025 per cent and 0.075 per cent capsaicin, rubbed in three or four times a day. Remember the effect builds up over time so don't get despondent if the first dose has only a mild effect. Keep on with it. For bloating, 0.25 grams of cayenne on the first mouthful of a meal would be about right. As regards the peppers themselves, their spiciness is measured in Scoville units. Jalapeño peppers vary between 2,500 and 8,000 Scoville units, while the bhut jolokia, recognized as the world's hottest chilli, reaches more than one million. The world record for eating bhut jolokias stands at over 50 in just two minutes but most people find it difficult to eat even one. A couple of average peppers should be enough to produce an analgesic effect.

▶ Any side effects?

There may be a stinging sensation lasting for up to two hours following the first few applications of capsaicin creams, but after a couple of days the stinging will stop. Do not use on broken or irritated skin. Eating a lot of chilli peppers may cause a burning sensation around the anus. In India, eating large and regular quantities of red chilli powder has been linked with an increased incidence of mouth and throat cancers.

CHIA SEEDS

▶ What will they do for me?

Chia seeds have recently become a 'superfood' in Europe but have been popular in the USA for a while. In South America their use dates back at least to the Aztecs. The Latin name is *Salvia hispanica*, a member of the mint family. The seeds are rich in omega-3 fatty acids, including a-linolenic acid (ALA). Perhaps their most useful effect is in protecting the stomach from acid, due to the way they triple in size in liquids to create a gelatinous and soothing gel.

▶ How should I use it?

Start with a sprinkling of seeds on a suitable dish such as muesli and work up from there. Never get full on a meal that includes chia because those chia seeds are going to expand – and that's going to be very uncomfortable.

▶ Any side effects?

Chia seeds are high in phytates which bind to minerals (such as iron, zinc and calcium) in the diet and either slow or prevent their absorption. Some nutritionists therefore describe chia as an 'anti-food'. However, that seems to be an exaggeration. All grains, legumes, nuts and seeds are high in phytates, yet vegetarians are not deficient.

COENZYME Q10 (ALSO KNOWN AS COQ10)

▶ What will it do for me?

Coenzyme Q10 is a vitamin-like substance that helps in the creation of adenosine triphosphate (ATP), the main power source in the body's cells. It is also an antioxidant. In one study, just over 60 per cent of migraine sufferers reported at least a 50 per cent reduction in the number of days they had headaches when taking CoQ10, and only 2 out of 32 showed no improvement at all.

▶ How should I use it?

Try 150 mg a day.

▶ Any side effects?

No serious side effects have been reported but a tiny minority of users have experienced nausea and diarrhoea.

DEVIL'S CLAW

▶ What will it do for me?

Devil's claw (*Harpagophytum procumbens*), also known as grapple plant, comes from South Africa. It is an anti-inflammatory that works, just as NSAIDs do, by inhibiting eicosanoids (messengers in the nervous system). It's been shown to be beneficial for those suffering from osteoarthritis of the knee and hip and also helps with chronic back pain.

▶ How should I use it?

Around 400 mg a day may be enough but some people take as much as 750 mg three times a day.

▶ Any side effects?

Don't take if you're on blood thinning medicines or are pregnant or breastfeeding or if you have liver or kidney disease or stomach ulcers.

DHEA

▶ What will it do for me?

DHEA (dehydroepiandrosterone) is a steroid hormone that peaks in the body in the mid-20s and declines to about one-fifth of that level by age 75. Numerous claims have been made for the rejuvenating effects of DHEA supplementation and Dr Norman Shealy, inventor of transcutaneous electrical nerve stimulation (TENS – see Chapter 10) promotes an acupuncture-based method of increasing DHEA as a cure for pain. However, although DHEA looks promising, there is as yet very little hard scientific evidence of any benefit from supplementation while, on the other hand, there are known side effects. It's available as a dietary supplement in the USA and on the internet in the UK.

▶ How should I use it?

DHEA supplements are prepared from yams. However, eating yams or yam products will not increase your DHEA as the human digestive system lacks the necessary enzyme. As a supplement, the standard DHEA dose is 25 – 50 mg a day.

▶ Any side effects?

Possible side effects include acne, hair loss, stomach upset, high blood pressure and, in women, facial hair, a deeper voice and changes in the menstrual cycle. Long-term side effects are not known. DHEA should not be taken by women who are pregnant or breastfeeding, or those with hormone-sensitive conditions or liver problems, and there may be drug interactions. Until more is known DHEA supplementation can't be recommended, but if all else has failed it's an option you could discuss with your doctor.

FEVERFEW (TANACETUM PARTHENIUM)

▶ What will it do for me?

Feverfew gets its name from the fact that it has long been used to treat fever. But it's also an effective preventative for migraine in about a quarter of people who suffer. That means, unfortunately, that three-quarters don't benefit at all, but you may be one of the lucky ones.

▶ How should I use it?

In one study, an effective dose for preventing migraines was found to be from 50 to 114 mg per day. You'll need to take feverfew every day and it will probably be a couple of weeks or so before you notice any benefit. If you choose to grow the plants, you'll need three small leaves (about 4 cm long) every day.

▶ Any side effects?

Some people have complained of mouth ulcers and skin irritations. Feverfew shouldn't be taken by women who are pregnant or breastfeeding. The Migraine Trust advises against taking it with NSAIDs. Stopping feverfew suddenly after the body has got used to it may cause a 'rebound' effect with migraines, anxiety, insomnia and nausea – if you decide to stop, taper over a few weeks.

GINGER

▶ What will it do for me?

Ginger (*Zingiber officinale*) has been used in China for more than 2,000 years to reduce inflammation (and, therefore, the pain that goes with it), treat digestive problems and combat nausea. It's extremely cunning. One of its actions is to block COX-2 enzymes but not COX-1, something that medical science has only recently achieved with the painkiller celecoxib (see Chapter 2). But while man-made COX-2-only inhibitors have serious side effects, ginger has almost none. The significance is this. NSAIDs such as ibuprofen inhibit COX-2 (thus reducing inflammation) but also COX-1, which normally protects the stomach. The result is that while NSAIDs can damage the stomach and cause bleeding, ginger does not.

Comparing ginger and NSAIDs in terms of pain control, one study found that, when used over a period of weeks, ginger was as effective as ibuprofen at reducing the joint pain caused by osteoarthritis. In another study, ginger provided significant pain relief to more than three-quarters of those who suffered from rheumatoid arthritis or osteoarthritis. And in a study at the University of Rochester Medical Center, headed by Julie L Ryan, those who took ginger supplements along with standard anti-vomiting drugs suffered 40 per cent less nausea following chemotherapy. (The ginger was given for three days prior to the treatment and for three days afterwards.)

▶ How should I use it?

If you're using fresh ginger you can simply peel a little of the rhizome and chew on it. You can also cut half a dozen thin slices from the rhizome to make an infusion with boiling water. In the form of tablets, up to around 500 mg of extract per day should be fine.

▶ Any side effects?

Some people are allergic to ginger and there have been cases in which it caused arrhythmia (irregular heartbeat), but the United States Food and Drug Administration (FDA) says ginger is 'generally recognized as safe'. Ginger has slight blood thinning properties and at doses above 500 mg per day may increase blood pressure.

GINKGO BILOBA

▶ What will it do for me?

Many benefits have been claimed for ginkgo biloba, prepared from the leaves of a tree that has been described as a 'living fossil', but science has rejected most of them. Among the conditions for which ginkgo does seem effective, however, is peripheral arterial disease (PAD) which can cause pain in various parts of the body and especially in the legs during exercise. A team of researchers supported by the respected National Centre for Complementary and Alternative Medicine (NCCAM) studied 3,069 men and women aged 75 and over, giving either a placebo or 120 mg of ginkgo twice daily over six years. Those on the ginkgo had fewer problems with PAD than those on placebo. An analysis of eight studies found that those on ginkgo could walk farther than those on placebo before experiencing pain. As a bonus, there's good evidence that ginkgo can give your sex life a boost by improving the circulation where it's most needed.

▶ How should I use it?

The standard dose is 120 mg once or twice a day.

▶ Any side effects?

Ginkgo has few side effects but some users have reported stomach upsets, skin reactions, dizziness and headaches. Ginkgo should not be taken with other medicaments as there could be an interaction; in particular it should never be taken with blood thinners. Do not take ginkgo if you are pregnant, breastfeeding, or have epilepsy or diabetes.

MAGNESIUM

▶ What will it do for me?

The human body contains a mere 24 grams of magnesium but it plays a vital role in various processes. Intriguingly, migraine sufferers seem to have low brain magnesium during attacks and there is at least some evidence that magnesium supplementation can help prevent them.

▶ How should I use it?

For the prevention of migraine take 600 mg daily for at least three months.

▶ Any side effects?

Some people have reported diarrhoea. There may be an interaction with antibiotics.

OMEGA-3 POLYUNSATURATED FATTY ACIDS

▶ What will they do for me?

In a study at the Pittsburgh Medical Center, 250 patients with nonsurgical back or neck pain were asked to take daily omega-3 polyunsaturated fatty acids (PUFAs) in the form of fish oil supplements. After one month all were sent a questionnaire. Half returned the questionnaire after an average of 75 days on the fish oil. Of those 125 patients, 78 per cent had been taking 1200 mg a day and 22 per cent had taken 2400 mg. The questionnaires showed that 59 per cent had discontinued taking their prescription NSAIDs, 60 per cent said their joint pain had diminished and the same percentage said their overall pain had gone down. No side effects were reported. This is exciting because it implies that omega-3s are as effective as NSAIDs for this type of problem, but without any of the drawbacks that can come with long-term NSAID use.

In addition to reducing inflammation (and, therefore, pain) omega-3s dilate blood vessels and deter blood platelets from sticking together, thus improving circulation. As a further bonus, there's evidence that omega-3s boost the mental performance of children in about 40 per cent of cases. One theory is that cell membranes high in omega-3 are more flexible and conduct brain signals more efficiently.

▶ How should I use it?

If you eat oily fish regularly you'll be getting enough. If not, you can take fish oil capsules. If you're a vegetarian or vegan then linseed (flaxseed) oil is your best choice, followed by rapeseed (canola), soy and walnut oil. However, there is a problem with vegetable sources of omega-3 because they contain only tiny amounts of two of the key nutrients, eicosapentaenoic acid (EPA) and decosahexaenoic acid (DHA). DHA is thought to be protective against rheumatoid arthritis as well as heart disease, blood pressure, arteriosclerosis, cardiac arrhythmias, anxiety, depression and, in the elderly, memory loss. EPA also eases depression and reduces heart disease. A study published in 2010 suggested that high levels of DHA/EPA might help maintain the length of telomeres on chromosomes, the shortening of which has been linked to ageing by some scientists.

Fortunately, the body can convert the main plant form of omega-3, alpha-linolenic acid (ALA), into DHA but at a rate that's believed to range from 20 per cent in young women to just 5 per cent in older men. The European Food Safety Authority recommends 250 mg of EPA/DHA a day, while the American Heart Association advises 500 mg. Allowing for the conversion, that means consuming between 1.25 g and 10 g of ALA per day. Given that linseed is roughly 50 per cent ALA, you'll need 2.5 – 20 grams (roughly a small teaspoon up to one and a half tablespoons) of linseed oil per person per day. That's easily done. Simply use linseed oil on bread or toast in place of butter or margarine, and in salad dressings. Don't cook with it.

▶ Any side effects?

Fish oil capsules may give you fishy breath. Taking more than 3 grams a day of fish oil may increase the risk of haemorrhage. If you're already prescribed blood thinners, consult your doctor before taking omega-3 supplements.

Remember this

All vegetable oils should be kept in the fridge once open (and stored in a dark place before opening), otherwise they oxidize. Oxidized oil is no longer beneficial – in fact, it's actually harmful – and this applies all the more so to linseed oil which oxidizes very rapidly. Buy small bottles you can use in about a week (for one person that would be 250 ml/9 fl oz).

QUERCETIN

▶ What will it do for me?

At the moment good scientific data is lacking but it seems to have anti-inflammatory properties and be beneficial in the treatment of fibromyalgia and prostatitis.

▶ How should I use it?

Quercetin occurs naturally in fruits, vegetables and grains, because it's a flavonoid or natural plant pigment. Red onions, kale and watercress contain particularly high amounts in proportion to weight but an apple is the easiest way, containing about 5 mg of quercetin. However, as a treatment for fibromyalgia you're going to need 300 mg – 500 mg a day, which can only be achieved through supplements, and as much as 500 mg twice daily has been used for the treatment of prostatitis for short periods.

▶ Any side effects?

No side effects are known from quercetin occurring naturally in food, but supplements have been known to cause headaches and tingling of the arms and legs. Doses higher than 1 gram per day risk kidney damage. Don't take quercetin supplements if you're pregnant or breastfeeding.

RESVERATROL

▶ What will it do for me?

Researchers at the University of Arizona found resveratrol (a substance in peanuts, certain fruits and especially the skins of red grapes) to be especially effective at reducing post-operative pain if injected at the sight of the incision. It also combats allodynia, a condition in which even a gentle touch becomes painful. By mouth, resveratrol has anti-inflammatory and antioxidant properties.

▶ How should I use it?

Although red wine contains resveratrol, the concentration is too low to be effective. Supplements are therefore the only way to self-medicate. The standard oral dose is 250 mg – 500 mg a day.

▶ Any side effects?

Studies have not yet found any severe side effects from resveratrol, other than an increased risk of bleeding if taken together with blood thinners such as warfarin, or with NSAIDs such as ibuprofen. However, some users have complained of joint and tendon pain while taking it.

SLIPPERY ELM

▶ What will it do for me?

Slippery elm (*Ulmus fulva* or *Ulmus rubra*) was used by Native Americans for a variety of problems including pain in the digestive system. It contains mucilage which becomes a gel when in contact with secretions in the digestive tract. It also stimulates the digestive tract to produce more mucous. It can therefore help reduce the pain of gastroesophageal reflux disease (GERD) and ulcers.

▶ How should I use it?

The easiest way to take slippery elm is as a tea. Half to one teaspoon of the powdered inner bark is enough for one cup. Drink around three cups a day. Alternatively, take around 250 – 400 mg in capsule form three times a day.

▶ Any side effects?

None have been recorded but, as a safety precaution, pregnant women should not take it. It may slow the absorption of other medicaments and therefore should be taken either two hours before them or two hours afterwards.

TURMERIC (CURCUMA LONGA)

▶ What will it do for me?

Turmeric is the yellow powder that contributes colour and flavour to curries. Part of the ginger family, its most important property is that it acts as an anti-inflammatory. In one experiment at the University of Arizona, the placebo effect was ruled out when turmeric was shown to inhibit joint swelling in rats. The key compound in turmeric seems to be curcumin, a powerful anti-oxidant. There is at least some evidence that turmeric may also fight fibromyalgia, certain infections, some cancers, heartburn, diarrhoea, gas, bloating, jaundice, and even depression and Alzheimer's disease.

▶ How should I use it?

You can simply eat lots of curry or use turmeric in other dishes. However, the best way to get a standardized dose is to take capsules of 500 mg two to four times a day. Unlike NSAIDs, the full anti-inflammatory effects will take a couple of weeks to develop, so wait a month before you decide whether or not turmeric works for you.

▶ Any side effects?

Turmeric is considered pretty safe but it's advised not to exceed 2,000 mg a day, nor to take turmeric while pregnant or breastfeeding. Don't take turmeric if you have gallstones or a bile duct obstruction. Surgeons recommend stopping turmeric two weeks before an operation, in case its blood-thinning properties increase bleeding. However, there are reports of faster post-operative recovery by patients who continue to take turmeric.

Case study

Nigel was a man in his early seventies who had been suffering with pain in both hips. His doctor prescribed NSAIDs which helped for a time. But when Nigel developed ulcers and could no longer tolerate NSAIDs he switched to turmeric tablets on the advice of a friend. Initially the turmeric seemed ineffective but after two weeks Nigel was almost free of pain and no longer walked with a limp.

VITAMIN B2 (RIBOFLAVIN)

▶ What will it do for me?

In one study of 55 migraine sufferers, 59 per cent reported at least a 50 per cent reduction in headaches when on vitamin B2 supplementation.

▶ How should I use it?

Vitamin B2 occurs naturally in lots of foods, especially leafy green vegetables, legumes, mushrooms, almonds, yeast, milk, cheese, liver and kidneys. In the study referred to above, sufferers took supplements of 400 mg a day for three months. The effect seems to be enhanced if riboflavin is taken together with magnesium and coenzyme Q10 (both of which are described above).

▶ Any side effects?

None at the recommended dose, but pregnant women are advised to discuss supplementation with their doctors. High doses of B2 turn urine a fluorescent yellow.

VITAMIN C

▶ What will it do for me?

Free radicals are known to be involved in the pain process. Vitamin C is an antioxidant which mops up free radicals and therefore reduces pain.

▶ How should I use it?

The typical Westerner consumes around 60 mg of vitamin C a day in food. Dr Robert Cathcart MD (1932–2007) described taking 12 grams every 15 minutes following a cornea transplant. 'By the time I reached 72 grams,' he says, 'there was absolutely no pain.' That's to say, in the space of 90 minutes he took more than one thousand times the normal daily dose, and 36 times the Tolerable Upper Intake Level (UL) specified by America's National Academy of Sciences. It's impossible to recommend such a regime but there's evidence that taking two grams a day, equivalent to the UL, may enhance the effect of whatever painkillers you're having.

▶ Any side effects?

Large doses of vitamin C can cause diarrhoea.

VITAMIN D

▶ What will it do for me?

If you're deficient in vitamin D you may experience pain in muscles and bones as well as fatigue. In one study, women experiencing musculoskeletal pain due to the action of anti-cancer drugs known as aromatase inhibitors gained considerable relief from weekly high-level doses of vitamin D. According to certain studies, low levels of vitamin D are associated with a higher risk of some cancers, diabetes, multiple sclerosis and heart disease.

▶ How should I use it?

Although there is some vitamin D in food (notably oily fish), the primary source is the action of sunlight on skin. That means many people are deficient in winter and, in the wetter parts of the globe, even in summer. North of 50 degrees (all of the UK and Canada) around half the population is thought to be deficient in winter because the intensity of the sunlight from

October to April is never sufficient. But in summer at that latitude three half-hour exposures to sunlight a week around the middle of the day should be enough. You don't have to lie in the sun in a swimming costume – having bare arms or legs will do. Never get sunburnt. For severe vitamin D deficiency kick start with a supplement of 2,000 iu (50 mcg) three times a day for five days only. After that, a sensible maintenance dose is 2,000 iu (50 mcg) a day in winter falling to 1,000 iu (25 mcg) in summer. In the study of women on aromatase inhibitors described above the dose was 50,000 iu (1,250 mcg) a week for 16 weeks, then monthly for two months.

▶ **Any side effects?**

The US National Academy of Sciences says the safe limit (known as the Tolerable Upper Intake Level) is 2,000 iu (50 mcg) a day but many scientists see no problem with even 10,000 iu (250 mcg). Intake of more than 50,000 iu (1,250 mcg) per day for several months has proven to be toxic.

Focus points

✻ Some foods are associated with painful inflammation while others can help reduce inflammation

✻ Some foods lead to blockages in the arteries while others can help clean arteries

✻ Some foods are associated with cancer while others can help reduce the risk

✻ Some foods can cause painful reactions, due to allergy or intolerance, and should be avoided

✻ Some foods can trigger migraine and need to be eliminated from the diet.

Next step

In the next chapter we'll be looking at something just as fundamental as food but a good deal more mysterious. It's the role of sleep – and relaxation – in sensitivity to pain.

Sleep therapy

> **In this chapter you will learn:**
>
> ▶ *how lack of sleep increases pain*
> ▶ *how meditation can help you*
> ▶ *how to get a good night's sleep.*

Among those experiencing chronic pain, about two-thirds report poor or unrefreshing sleep.

National Sleep Foundation, USA.

In the UK about 35 per cent of adults are believed to suffer from insomnia although only about 5 per cent consult their doctors. If you're in pain you're very likely to be one of them. Monitoring bodily functions during sleep (a technique known as polysomnography or PSG) clearly shows that acute pain leads to shortened and fragmented sleep, with reduced amounts of slow wave and REM ('dreaming') sleep. In chronic pain the impact on sleep is less severe, probably because sufferers learn to adjust to some extent.

It also works the other way around. Shortened or fragmented sleep heightens the perception of pain. Researchers from the Division of Rheumatology and Pain Management Centre of Brigham and Women's Hospital together with the Chronic Pain and Fatigue Center of the University of Michigan Medical School, investigated 59 women with rheumatoid arthritis (RA) and found that sleep problems were inversely associated with pain thresholds both in the joints and elsewhere in the body. In other words, limited or disturbed sleep increases the sensation of pain throughout the body.

And it's not only about pain. In a study led by Dr Faith S Luyster at the University of Pittsburgh School of Nursing, poor sleep quality also correlated with fatigue and greater functional disability.

It's a circle. Poor sleep leads to a whole package of problems which in turn makes it harder to sleep.

? Diagnostic test

Let's take a look at how you're doing at the moment. Score one point for every statement you agree with. You may choose more than one statement for each of the ten topics below.

1 I (a) take a long time to fall asleep (b) wake up several times a night (c) still feel tired in the morning.

2 I get headaches (a) most weeks (b) at weekends but seldom during the working week (c) in clusters.

3 I often have (a) butterflies in my stomach (b) unusual hair loss (c) nosebleeds.

4 I find my problems (a) frightening (b) insurmountable (c) growing and growing.

5 I (a) grind my teeth (b) bite my nails (c) find it difficult to keep still.

6 As regards sex, with a partner or alone (a) I can't even think about it (b) I try but I'm not very responsive (c) it's painful.

7 I'm dependent on (a) comfort eating (b) cigarettes (c) alcohol (d) drugs, other than those prescribed for my condition.

8 I (a) find it hard to make decisions (b) neglect things I know I should be doing.

9 I often feel (a) agitated (b) irritable (c) angry.

10 I (a) seem to catch every bug that's going around (b) need antibiotics several times a year.

▶ **Your score**

▶ If you scored 20 or over you're dangerously stressed and sleep-deprived. You need to take urgent action. If your stress is due to your pain, hopefully this book can help but if it's partly due to your lifestyle you need to make serious changes, starting right now.

▶ If you scored 13 to 19 you're highly stressed and the quality of your sleep is probably poor. If your stress is due to your pain, hopefully this book can help but if it's partly due to your lifestyle you should seriously think about the changes you need to make and implement them step by step.

▶ If you scored 6 to 12, you're probably average but that's not good enough.

▶ If you scored one to five you're obviously a pretty laid-back person with a relaxed lifestyle but you may still learn a few useful things from this chapter.

▶ If you scored zero you're not stressed or sleep-deprived at all and you can skip this chapter if you like.

How much sleep do I need?

The accepted wisdom is that most adults need seven to eight hours of sleep a night but everyone is different. The Epworth Sleepiness Scale below gives a good indication of whether or not you're getting enough sleep for you.

For each of the following score 0 if you have no chance of dozing, 1 if there's a slight chance of dozing, 2 if there's a moderate chance of dozing, and 3 if there's a high chance of dozing.

1 Sitting and reading

2 Watching TV

3 Sitting inactive in a public place (such as a theatre or a meeting)

4 As a passenger in a car for an hour without a break

5 Lying down to rest in the afternoon when circumstances permit

6 Sitting and talking to someone

7 Sitting quietly after a lunch without alcohol

8 In a car, while stopped for a few minutes in traffic.

Add up all your points. If you scored zero to six you're getting enough sleep. If you scored seven to eight you're not getting quite enough but you're nevertheless about average. If you scored nine or over you need to study this chapter very carefully.

Key idea

A study published in the journal Sleep in 2012 found that people who typically slept for 10 hours a night were able to endure pain for 25 seconds longer than those who slept eight hours or less.

Remember this

Sleep is divided into two main types. Rapid Eye Movement (REM) sleep and non-REM sleep. Non-REM sleep is further divided into four stages:

✳ Stage 1 – drowsiness
✳ Stage 2 – light sleep
✳ Stages 3 and 4 – deep or slow-wave sleep.

First learn to relax

In order to sleep you first have to relax. Relaxation is itself an analgesic. In one study, patients undergoing colorectal surgery who listened to guided imagery relaxation tapes before, after, and even during surgery, needed fewer painkillers than those who did not. Apart from easing pain generally, relaxation will improve symptoms in a number of painful conditions, including:

▶ Fibromyalgia

▶ Chronic tension headaches

▶ Arthritis

▶ Irritable Bowel Syndrome.

Key idea

According to the Mind/Body Institute at Harvard University 60 – 90 per cent of all consultations with a doctor in the USA are related to stress. So stress is an extremely dangerous thing. You need to avoid it.

BREATH CONTROL

Have you noticed that when you feel tense or frightened you tend to hold your breath? And when you do breathe you do so with short, constricted movements? It's nature's way of making you less obvious to predators. And because of that it's also linked with hormonal changes connected with the 'fight or flight' response, especially the stress hormone cortisol. You get trapped in a cycle in which tension affects your breathing and your breathing perpetuates your tension.

The way to break that cycle is to consciously take control of your breathing for a while. You need to make it:

▶ Slower

▶ From the belly

▶ With exhalations 50 per cent longer than inhalations.

By doing so you'll force your body to go into relaxation mode which, in turn, will ease a variety of pains.

Try it now

Here's what to do:

1 Place your left hand on your heart and your right hand on your stomach immediately below your navel
2 Inhale for a count of seven, feeling your stomach rise
3 Hold for a count of two
4 Exhale for a count of 11, feeling your stomach deflate
5 Pause for a count of four
6 Repeat the whole cycle again and again for at least four minutes.

Initially you may feel a bit breathless as you try to get the length of your inhalations and exhalations right but after a minute or so you should be able to find a timing that you can easily maintain. From that point on you should feel increasingly relaxed.

RELAXING MUSCLES

Here's an exercise to relax your body. If you sleep with a partner, he or she will have to be very understanding or sneak into bed after you've dropped off.

Try it now

1 Lie in bed on your back with your arms a little away from your sides, palms upwards, and your legs comfortably apart.
2 While breathing in, clench your right fist, contract the muscles in your right arm and raise it a few inches; breathe out and let your arm flop back down.

3 Do the same with your left arm.

4 While breathing in, turn your right foot back towards your knee so your calf muscle is stretched (i.e. the opposite of pointing your toes) and raise your leg a few inches; breathe out and let it flop back down.

5 Do the same with your left leg.

6 Whilst breathing out visualize your trunk and head sagging and sinking into the bed, which supports and embraces you like warm water.

7 Whilst breathing out visualize your arms and legs sinking into the bed, which supports and embraces you like warm water.

Repeat the whole cycle over and over until you feel relaxed. If you don't feel relaxed after 10 minutes switch to another strategy.

Remember this

Paradoxical as it may seem, that relaxing Sunday lie-in can sometimes be a source of pain, especially headaches. If you have a high-speed, very stressful life from Monday to Saturday then the sudden change in hormones and neurotransmitters precipitated by 'snoozy Sunday' can make you feel really ill. The best solution is to aim for a less stressful lifestyle. If that isn't possible, at least try to fit in some daily relaxation. If you fail to do even that then you'd better get up on Sunday at the same time as the rest of the week.

Drugs and insomnia

Unfortunately, some medicaments, including painkillers, can interfere with sleep. If you never used to have sleep problems before you started taking them then they're the first things to suspect. Read about side effects in the leaflets accompanying the drugs and discuss alternatives with your doctor. Here are the main culprits:

▶ Analgesics. Painkillers that contain caffeine should be avoided. The best alternative in terms of sleep quality seems to be paracetamol on its own. Some studies have found ibuprofen detrimental to sleep but at least one other didn't.

As regards something stronger, a study by the Pain Centre of Fairfield in the USA concluded that opioids were beneficial for sleep. In another study, opiods decreased both slow-wave and REM sleep, yet patients subjectively reported their quality of sleep was better. It seems the effects are very individual and you may need to experiment to find the most suitable analgesic for you.

► Antidepressants. Although antidepressants are often prescribed for insomnia they can also suppress REM sleep, increase the number of awakenings, and decrease total sleep time. Antidepressants may also exacerbate restless leg syndrome. If you suspect antidepressants may be causing you sleep problems, speak to your doctor about an alternative kind.

► Decongestants

► Cough medicines

► The herbal remedies St John's wort, ginseng and Sam-e

► Medications for attention-deficit hyperactivity disorder (ADHD)

► Nicotine patches

► Antidepressants of the class known as selective serotonin reuptake inhibitors (SSRIs)

► Cholesterol-lowering drugs

► Drugs for lowering high blood pressure

► Drugs for controlling heart arrhythmias.

Your doctor may advise a substitute medicine or simply changing the time of day at which you take the existing medicine.

Meditation for sleep and pain relief

A great deal of mystique surrounds meditation involving gurus and special 'mantras' but, in fact, it's something perfectly straightforward that everyone can do. There are various different styles of meditation. What we're interested in here is achieving an increased degree of control over your mind, both conscious and unconscious, so you can reduce your pain and become relaxed enough to fall asleep.

In meditation you will enter a state of consciousness which is neither the normal, everyday state of being awake nor of being asleep. Broadly there are four categories of brainwaves of which two are associated with meditation:

1 Beta: 13 – 40 Hz. The fastest frequencies associated with normal waking consciousness and being alert.

2 Alpha: 7 – 13 Hz. The next fastest frequencies, associated with feeling relaxed, daydreaming, reverie and light meditation.

3 Theta: 4 – 7 Hz. Slower again, associated with dreaming sleep and deep meditation.

4 Delta: Under 4 Hz. The slowest, associated with deep sleep.

Note the use of the word 'associated' because, in fact, it's possible for two, three, or even four frequencies to be present at the same time. Although light meditation is normally said to be in alpha mode and deep meditation in theta mode, in practice deep meditation can involve not just theta but also beta and, in rare cases, all four. That is normally the preserve of a 'master' possessing what's known as an 'awakened mind'. When you meditate you'll certainly combine frequencies in a way that's different to sleeping.

So let's get started.

The first thing to sort out is a time and place to meditate. As I'm suggesting you use meditation to help you get off to sleep then it makes sense to meditate at bedtime. But if you enjoy it there's no reason you shouldn't also meditate at other times – perhaps first thing in the morning or when you get home after work. As to the place, the bed itself is fine. Turn the light out or wear an eye mask of some sort to minimize distractions.

We've all seen pictures of people meditating in the lotus position but that certainly isn't essential and, indeed, for most people it's impossible. I would suggest you begin by sitting up on the bed with your feet pulled up towards your buttocks (it's not necessary to cross your ankles if you find it uncomfortable). Have some pillows to support your back and another under the rear of your buttocks to tip your pelvis slightly forwards. If your pain prevents you from sitting up on the bed like this you can sit on the edge of the bed with your feet on the floor. Once you're close to a meditative state I'm going to suggest that you then lie down flat on top of the bed.

Different people use different techniques, ranging from the chanting of a mantra to staring at a candle but I'm going to give you a method here that's easy and works for most people.

Try it now

1 In your chosen position smile (just a 'secret' little smile will do).

2 Gradually slow down your breathing, making sure your stomach rises as you breathe in, and descends as you breathe out.

3 Regulate your breathing. Inhale through your nose for a count of 7, hold for a count of 2, exhale through your mouth for a count of 11, pause for a count of 4, then inhale for a count of 7 again. Continue like that, focusing on your breathing and counting. Everyday thoughts and worries will try to intrude. If they do, don't pursue them. Just let them go and get back to your counting.

4 While you're breathing in (and counting up to 7) move the ring finger of your left hand against the fleshy base of your thumb. While you're breathing out (and counting up to 11) move your ring finger away again.

5 When you're breathing is slow and relaxed and you're little bothered by intrusive thoughts you can stop counting and instead focus on your heartbeat. Once you can 'hear' it, try to think it slower. Keep the finger movement going in time with your breath.

6 Notice the sound of blood pulsing in your left ear. If you can't detect it, try swivelling your closed eyes to the left. Try thinking the pulse slower.

7 Notice the sound of blood pulsing in your right ear. If you can't detect it, try swivelling your closed eyes to the right. Try thinking the pulse slower.

8 If you haven't already done so, lie down flat on your back on the bed, your legs slightly apart and your arms a little away from your sides, palms up. Continue to feel very relaxed. Notice the little white dots that illuminate the blackness of your closed eyes like stars in the sky. Choose one of the 'stars' and head towards it.

9 By this stage images may appear from out of nowhere. You may see faces of people that, as far as you know, you've

never met or even seen. This is a sign that you're reaching a meditative state.

10 As you continue to 'follow that star' and go deeper still, you'll become intensely aware of the functioning of your body – breathing, heart, blood flow. Your lips and fingers may feel as if they're swollen and heavy.

11 Next you may feel as if you're coming out of the meditative state without intending to. You feel alert although 'spaced out' and somewhat detached. If you reach this stage, resist the temptation to stop because it presages entry into an even deeper meditative state.

12 You now feel at one with the universe. Nothing seems to matter. You feel light and calm.

Key idea

When you begin meditating you're unlikely to reach the deepest level for some weeks. Be patient. It will take a while for your brain to adapt. But the more often you practise, the more readily you'll slip into a meditative state. If you can reach stage 10 after a week then you're doing well. That would be a good moment to slide beneath the covers and fall asleep. Stage 12 might take months.

Case study

'A friend suggested I try meditation and it's definitely helped me. When I got into bed at night I used to be especially conscious of my joint pain and I'd lie there desperately trying to go to sleep but all the time worrying about the future and what was going to become of me. Meditation has given me more control of my mind. I do it at bedtime. As a result, I've stopped rehearsing the same old thoughts over and over again. I feel calmer and I drift off to sleep more easily. When I wake up in the morning I feel more relaxed and it seems to take less time to get moving.' Wendy (57)

Tips for falling asleep

Sometimes quite small things can stop you falling asleep or wake you in the middle of the night. Here are some ideas to help you.

- During the daytime try to get in some vigorous exercise so that by bedtime both your body and your brain are tired.

- Worries always seem worse at night. So do your best in the daytime to deal with any anxieties you may have and to find solutions for problems. When you go to bed say this to yourself: 'Today I did everything possible to deal with my problems. I can now go to sleep knowing that nothing more could be done. Tomorrow I will awake refreshed and ready to tackle my problems again.'

- Don't finish a large meal within a couple of hours of going to bed, especially not a meal that's high in protein.

- Eat carbohydrate-rich foods for your evening meal (such as pasta, rice or potatoes) because they will cause the release of serotonin, a neurotransmitter that will help you sleep.

- Don't drink much alcohol in the evening. It's relaxing initially but in the body it becomes converted to acetaldehyde which is a stimulant. What's more, alcohol may cause dehydration. These two things together will wake you up in the early hours.

- Don't drink caffeine in the evening because it's a stimulant. It's contained in coffee (especially coffee prepared directly from coffee beans), tea, cola, energy drinks, and chocolate for eating (as a drink, hot chocolate contains very little caffeine).

- Don't watch disturbing television programmes before bedtime.

- Make sure it's neither too hot nor too cold in the bedroom and that the covers are neither too heavy nor too flimsy.

- If you sleep in a double bed with a restless partner consider getting single beds.

- When you're in bed, think of something that's both very nice and very engrossing. It doesn't have to be a real thing. It could be a fantasy. As you're lying there, 'play' the 'film' in your mind. If it's compelling enough it should crowd out worrying thoughts.

- If you have a partner, sex at bedtime can be a great 'sleeping pill' (see below). If you don't have a partner, solo sex will help in the same way.

Sex for relaxation, analgesia and sleep

Sex is a great tonic. It relaxes you. It's a mild painkiller. And it helps you to sleep. So sex at bedtime is a very good idea. But is it possible to have it for long enough and often enough to really make a difference to your life? Yes, it is. What follows is written with the heterosexual couple in mind. But the underlying science equally applies to same sex couples and to people on their own.

Key idea

Sex produces various chemical changes in the body including:

* An increase in dopamine which gets into the frontal lobe of the brain in the build-up to orgasm and during orgasm itself, producing a feeling of bliss and dulling feelings of pain.
* An increase in PEA (Phenylethylamine), an amphetamine-like substance that gives you a 'walking on air' kind of feeling.

The longer sex goes on, within reason, the greater the chemical changes.

Case study

'I suffer a lot with headaches. If I have a bad one then, of course, I can't contemplate sex. But if I feel a headache just starting to come on and I then have sex it's a different story. Nine times out of ten the headache goes away.' Tania (36)

PROLONGING SEX

When the famous sexologist Alfred Kinsey (1894–1956) was doing his research in America in the 1940s, he discovered that on half the occasions heterosexual couples had sex, men ejaculated within two minutes. Nowadays, research suggests men do better but still not well enough. A quickie may help a man (because ejaculation releases a chemical called prolactin, which we'll learn more about in a moment) but it won't do much for a woman. So the first requirement is for the man to be able to prolong intercourse for at least 15 minutes. Longer would be better. That way you'll both be full of dopamine and PEA.

Various ways of controlling ejaculation have been put forward by sexologists and sex gurus. Some require months of training, some are painful, and some don't work. But there is a simple system that most men can master quite quickly.

The crucial first step is for you, the man, to change your mental attitude. Stop seeing ejaculation as the whole point of sex. Instead, see it as failure. Why? Because ejaculation brings a man's chemical production line grinding to a halt. For pain relief (for either or both of you), you want to keep those chemical factories operating.

Rather than focus on ejaculation, focus instead on all the other delightful aspects of sex. Tell yourself that, no matter what happens, you will not ejaculate for, say, a quarter of an hour.

Having got that goal firmly in your mind, the next step is to practise on your own. Arouse yourself in your usual way and each time you approach the 'point of no return' (PNR) stop all forms of stimulation:

▶ Stop rubbing

▶ Stop fantasizing (if you were)

▶ Stop looking at sexy images (if you were)

▶ Stop 'talking dirty' (if you were)

▶ Stop concentrating on the sensations.

Initially, don't get too close to the PNR because, obviously, the closer you get the harder it becomes to retain control. But once you're able to keep self-stimulation going for a while you're ready to get closer to the PNR using the more sophisticated techniques described below.

▶ Breathing techniques for ejaculation control

Whilst stimulating yourself, breathe slowly and deeply. Make your exhalation about 50 per cent longer than your inhalation.

When you're in danger of going beyond the PNR, however, your breathing tactics will need to change. Stick your tongue out and down and exhale as forcefully as you can. Keep doing it, panting like a mad dog, until the urge to ejaculate has passed.

An alternative technique is to inhale in short bursts, while at the same time sucking your stomach inwards, and visualizing energy being drawn away from your penis and up your spine into your brain.

▶ The locking method

The final weapon in the ejaculation-control armoury is the locking method. First described by physicians of the Chinese Taoist religion thousands of years ago, it consists of simultaneously contracting the PC and abdominal muscles so that the stomach is pulled back towards the spine as far as possible.

The PC is the popular name for the muscle you use to hold back when you feel the urge to pee but there's nowhere to go. Strengthening it is vital to ejaculation control. You can flex it easily and invisibly whether standing or sitting, which means you can exercise it at any time. A basic exercise is to contract the muscle, hold for one or two seconds, then release. Repeat ten times several times a day. Once you can do that you're ready to move on to more advanced exercises:

▶ Contract and release your PC muscle rapidly for ten seconds. Repeat as many times as possible with breaks of ten seconds in between.

▶ After warming up with the previous exercise, contract and hold the PC muscle, initially for 30 seconds increasing to 2 minutes as your strength improves. Rest and repeat five times.

▶ Contract the PC muscle in five stages, holding each intermediate stage for 5 seconds and the maximum contraction for 30 seconds.

You can combine the locking method with the panting method for maximum control.

Remember this

Not only will a strong PC muscle improve your control but it will also increase the power of your ejaculations and enable you to flex your penis inside your partner's vagina, which should feel very nice for her. So it's well worth spending a few minutes a day on this.

▶ Practising with your partner

Having sex with a partner complicates things. It's relatively easy for you, the man, to cease stimulation but your partner also has to cease at exactly the same moment and wait until the danger of going beyond the PNR has receded. You could have an agreed verbal signal ('stop') but a less disruptive and more romantic way of going about things is to use a physical signal, such as holding her hips still. As time goes by you'll get better and better at 'reading' one another and slow down or speed up accordingly.

▶ To ejaculate or not to ejaculate?

So you now know how to prolong sex and build up those beneficial chemicals. But how can you have sex often enough to make a real difference? It's not a problem for a woman alone (or with another woman). But it is a problem for a woman and a man because most men aren't capable of daily sex. And even those men who can have daily sex may run into a problem with a chemical called prolactin.

Prolactin is a bit of a double-edged sword. It peaks at ejaculation and makes men feel fatigued. That's why men often fall asleep after sex, which for a man in pain is one of the main points of the whole exercise. But it also tends to make men slightly depressed (the so-called 'sexual hangover') and the effect can last a considerable time. That's the opposite of what you need when you're already in pain and anxious.

Prolactin is also the chemical that makes it impossible to have sex again for a time. For a young man the 'refractory period' during which sex is impossible might be seconds or minutes but for an older man prolactin, acting with other changes in the body, can make it hours or days.

So if you're aiming to use sex as a daily tonic you need to think carefully about ejaculation. (For women things are slightly different – prolactin is produced throughout sex, rather than peaking at orgasm, but in smaller, less potent, quantities.)

The solution to the conundrum is for the man to have sex without ejaculating, at least some of the time. Daily sex then becomes quite possible. And if you carry on having sex for long enough you'll both be happily tired anyway.

If you'd like to learn more about these techniques you'll find a full explanation in *Have Great Sex* and *Get Intimate With Tantric Sex* in the Teach Yourself series.

🔑 Key idea

If you want to use sex as a 'medicine' in this way then it's something you need to discuss quite openly with your partner (unless you're going to have sex on your own). Explain that you'd like to try daily sex as a relaxant, painkiller and 'sleeping pill' and ask for his or her co-operation. You both need to be in agreement on this.

❗ Focus points

* When you're in pain you can't sleep normally
* When you can't sleep your sensitivity to pain increases
* Some medicaments, including analgesics, can interfere with sleep
* Relaxation techniques such as breath control and meditation can put you in the mood for sleep
* Sex can act as an analgesic and 'sleeping potion'.

➡ Next step

Sex isn't an appropriate painkiller for everyone. But there are some other very nice things you can do physically. In the next chapter we'll be looking at, among other things, massages, hot water bottles and infrared lamps.

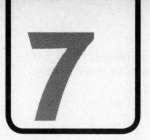

Massage therapy

In this chapter you will learn:

▶ *how massage works at the genetic level*
▶ *how you can give yourself an effective massage*
▶ *how heat can be as effective as a painkilling tablet.*

When we honestly ask ourselves which person in our lives means the most to us, we often find that it is those who, instead of giving advice, solutions, or cures, have chosen rather to share our pain and touch our wounds with a warm and tender hand.

Henri Nouwen, Catholic priest and writer (1932–1996)

Touch is very important to human beings. Babies and infants who, for whatever reason, experience little or no cuddling, fail to develop normally and may die, even if all their other needs are met. When we're feeling low or ill, a friendly touch always makes us feel at least a little bit better.

We all also instinctively touch ourselves where we feel pain or discomfort. When we were children mummy 'kissed it better', and as adults we rub our eyes, scratch the tops of our heads, squeeze the backs of our necks and massage banged knees. We stand by a fire or lie in the sun to relax our muscles.

But can massage really achieve very much beyond being a distraction? Is heat anything more than a pleasant sensation? Could it be possible to manipulate another person's energies simple by bringing hands close, without actually touching? Can the insertion of needles into the body achieve more than the techniques used at the body's surface?

These are some of the questions I'll be looking at and answering in this chapter. But, first of all, here are some questions for you.

Diagnostic test

1 Are your painkillers causing unpleasant side effects?

2 Are your painkillers less effective than they used to be?

3 Are you experiencing pain despite the medications you're taking?

4 Have you had to increase the strength of your painkillers?

5 Do you feel that your existing treatment needs topping up?

6 Are you open-minded about alternative therapies?

7 Are you comfortable with the idea of a stranger touching your body?

8 Do you find that touch is important to you?

9 Have you ever found that rubbing in a particular way or pressing hard on a particular point has reduced your pain?

10 Would you like to take control of your treatment?

▶ **Your score**

If you answered 'yes' to most questions then touch therapies should suit you very well. Touch therapies generally require a professional therapist but if you answered 'yes' to question 10 you'll be pleased to know there are also certain things you can do for yourself. Which are the best touch therapies? Read on.

The benefits of massage

Possibly you've already had a professional massage or, maybe, you've been given a massage by your partner. For sure you've often given yourself a massage when you had an ache and could reach it. But can massage really go beyond 'nice' and be a serious treatment for pain? Can it genuinely reduce it or even cure you completely?

The surprising answer is that it can.

THE EVIDENCE FOR MASSAGE

In a trial by the Center for Health Studies in Seattle, patients with persistent back pain were given up to ten weekly massage sessions. At the end of the 10-week period the massaged patients had fewer symptoms and greater mobility than similar patients on 'self care'. They also used fewer medications.

At least two studies have found massage effective in reducing pain specifically in cancer patients and at least two studies have also found it effective for relieving the pain of tension headaches.

Massage can also help in other ways. A study published in the Journal of Alternative and Complementary Medicine in September 2010 revealed that a single deep-tissue 'Swedish' massage caused a significant decrease in a hormone known as arginine vasopressin (AVP) which causes contraction of the blood vessels and a rise in blood pressure. The researchers found evidence that massage also reduces the stress hormone cortisol, and increases cancer-fighting white blood cells known as lymphocytes. And several studies have found that anxiety, which can cause various painful conditions, is reduced by massage.

Remember this

As long as the person giving the massage – a professional therapist, your partner, or you yourself – is considerate and doesn't cause pain, it's difficult to do any harm with massage. So you've got nothing to lose by giving it a go.

HOW DOES MASSAGE WORK?

Although massage is a natural instinct and has been around for thousands of years, the way it works is still not fully understood.

One theory, championed by Janet G. Travell (1901–1997), who worked on President John F. Kennedy's back problems, is that 'trigger points' (also called myofascial trigger points) develop within the muscles through overexertion.

When you move, individual microscopic sections of muscle fibres, known as sarcomeres, expand or contract. A single muscle cell might contain as many as 100,000 sarcomeres and a movement would involve billions of sarcomeres. Normally sarcomeres expand and contract like tiny pumps, but when they become frozen in the contracted position, so blood flow stops, waste products accumulate and oxygen starvation occurs. The result is pain.

Janet Travell wrote a book, together with David Simons, (*Myofascial Pain and Dysfunction: The Trigger Point Manual*) in which they argued that trigger points were the primary cause of pain in three-quarters of musculoskeletal problems and that they were almost always involved to a degree. You could have herniated discs and arthritis, for example, and yet myofascial trigger points could still be the primary cause of your back pain.

But here's a curious thing. The pain isn't normally felt at the site of the contracted sarcomeres but is 'referred' to another part of the body. For example, a diagonal shooting chest pain might be cured by massaging a trigger point in the neck. Sinus pain might be ended by massaging muscles in the jaw. And foot pain might be treated by massaging the calf muscle.

Massage, Travell and Simons argued, flushed blood through the trigger points and released the sarcomeres. Trigger point massage, they said, would cure most problems in three to ten days although chronic conditions might require six weeks.

One of Janet's sayings was: 'Life is like a bicycle – you don't fall off until you stop pedalling. It is better to wear out than to rust out, so keep pedalling.' She seems to have followed her own advice and didn't fall off the bicycle until she was 96.

Key idea

Given the phenomenon of referred pain it may be better to opt for a whole body massage rather than to focus on the place it hurts – the real problem may lie elsewhere and the whole body massage should then pick it up.

It seems, however, that massage may work in a way far more profound than even Janet Travell imagined. A team led by Mark Tarnopolsky at McMaster University in Hamilton, Ontario, recruited 11 young men as guinea pigs and subjected them to a gruelling cycling session. Afterwards, one leg was given a massage but the other was left to recover on its own. When the scientists compared the biopsies taken from the volunteers' quadriceps muscles before and after exercise, the results were astonishing. The massaged legs had 30 per cent more of a gene called PGC-1alpha which helps build mitrochondria, the 'power stations' in cells. The massaged legs also had three times less NFkB, which turns on genes linked to inflammation.

In other words, massage actually works at the genetic level to reduce inflammation and, therefore, pain.

Remember this

In a survey conducted for the American Massage Therapy Association (AMTA), about a fifth of Americans had had a massage in the previous year. Of those, 28 per cent said massage gave them 'the greatest relief from pain', a result that was on a par with medication.

BOOKING A PROFESSIONAL MASSAGE

In the UK there is no single organization that regulates the massage profession, nor are massage therapists required by law to be members of any particular body, nor is there a legal requirement to have completed any specific training. The best advice is to choose only therapists who belong to member organizations of the General Council for Massage Therapies (GCMT) which acts as an umbrella body. In the USA, the American Massage Therapy Association (AMTA) is the largest non-profit, professional association representing massage therapy and was founded in 1943. AMTA recommends a minimum of 500 hours of supervised in-class initial massage therapy training, which must include the study of anatomy and physiology. Most states license massage therapists, meaning that it would be illegal to work without a licence. There is a national certification administered by the National Certification Board for Therapeutic Massage and Bodywork (NCBTMB). (Contact details for GCMT and AMTA can be found in the Bibliography at the end of the book.)

Having drawn up a list of convenient, qualified therapists, the next task is to find out what kind of massage they offer. It could be:

► Swedish massage

► Thai massage

► Chinese massage

► Therapeutic massage

► Remedial massage

► Sports massage

► Myofascial massage

► Hot stone massage

► Trigger point massage

► NeuroDynamic massage

► DermoNeuroModulation

► Myotherapy.

In reality, an experienced therapist should be 'integrated', that's to say, skilled in a number of these disciplines. As a newcomer, avoid therapists who only offer one thing. Instead, favour those who can vary their approach and leave it to them to decide what's most appropriate in your case.

If you have mobility problems associated with your pain you may prefer a physiotherapist (or physical therapist) who, in addition to massage, will have a whole package of other techniques available including acupuncture (see below), exercise (Chapter 8), and transcutaneous electrical nerve stimulation (TENS) and ultrasound (see Chapter 10 for these two)

Do:

▶ Make a shortlist of three therapists and have one session with each of them before deciding who you'll stick with

▶ Make sure they've been practising as professionals for at least a year

▶ Make sure they have experience of dealing with your specific problem

▶ Make your final decision on the basis of who most investigated your medical history, gave you treatment most tailored to your problem and reduced your pain immediately and for a good while afterwards.

Don't:

▶ Continue with a treatment that's painful

▶ Stick with a therapist who tries to pressure you into a series of treatments

▶ Be taken in by talk of auras, balancing chakras or anything of that sort – favour those who follow a scientific approach.

▶ Warning

Massage isn't appropriate for everyone. Speak to your doctor first if you're pregnant or you have:

▶ Fractures or severe osteoporosis

▶ Rheumatoid arthritis

- Cancer
- Open wounds or burns
- Blood clots.

PARTNER MASSAGE

Can a massage by someone without formal training actually be of much use in reducing pain? Yes, it can. And here's the proof.

A study funded by the National Center for Alternative and Complementary Medicine and published in the Annals of Internal Medicine followed 400 people with chronic back pain. They were randomly divided into three groups. One group had 10 weeks of whole body massage for general relaxation, one had 10 weeks of massage targeted on specific muscles, and the third had 'usual care' (which covered a variety of treatments, from painkillers and muscle relaxants to chiropractors or, in some cases, nothing at all).

At the end of the 10 week period, only 4 per cent of the 'usual care' group said their pain was nearly or completely gone, compared with 36 per cent of the general massage group and 39 per cent of the specific muscle group. Now, what's significant here is that general massage was almost as effective as targeted massage. And general massage for relaxation is something your partner can learn to do for you.

The subject of massage needs a book on its own. Better still, I recommend you and your partner take a short course, say a weekend, to properly understand how it's done. Meanwhile, here are some ideas to help your partner get started (and there's no reason you shouldn't return the favour, even if your partner is pain-free).

A bed is too soft for a good massage. A folded blanket on the floor is much better. You'll need some kind of massage oil. There's no need to spend a lot of money on it. A light oil from the kitchen, such as soya, grapeseed or almond, will do perfectly well. Warm the oil first.

The general principle is to work inwards from the hands and feet and upwards from the base of the spine. Ask your partner to tell you what feels good and what doesn't.

Here are the basic techniques:

▶ Effleurage is a French word denoting a soothing, stroking action. Try it on the back to begin with. Your partner should be lying face down, head turned sideways and arms at the sides. With your hands covered in warm massage oil, put one hand each side of your partner's spine and push steadily up to the neck, keeping the whole surface of your hands and fingers in contact. When you arrive at the neck, continue out along the shoulders and then, with very light pressure only, glide your hands back down along your partner's sides to the starting position. Repeat several times.

▶ Kneading is a technique to use on tense muscles. The shoulders are a great place to start. At the end of effleurage, move both hands to one shoulder, pick up the muscle in one hand, squeeze it gently, then push it towards the other hand. The new hand then also kneads the muscle before pushing it back. In this way, the muscle is worked rhythmically between the two hands. Once you've done one shoulder, turn your attention to the other.

▶ Two fingers (the pads of your index and middle fingers) can be used to make small circular movements. Work your way up from the base of the spine to the neck, doing both sides simultaneously. You can also work on the muscles in this way.

Try it now

Ask your partner to get to work on you right away, somewhere that's useful and easily accessible – perhaps your shoulders or your calves. Ask him or her to try to sense the 'areas of contraction' and massage them away.

Key idea

It's important to realize that muscles are not smooth. Just because something feels uneven doesn't mean it's an 'area of contraction' (or what's popularly but inaccurately referred to as a 'knot'). An irregularity may, in fact, be perfectly normal. Only with time and patience can your partner learn to tell the difference.

Self-massage techniques

If you don't have anyone to give you a massage you can still get many of the benefits by massaging yourself. Unless you have mobility problems you should be able to reach your legs, feet and head, work one-handed on each arm, massage your abdomen, and do a little bit of useful work on your neck and shoulders as well as part of your back. But what about the places you can barely reach? In fact, with a little cunning you can even massage them – as you'll see in a moment. Here, then, are some self-massage ideas.

▶ The whole body pummel

Using your right fist, gently thump your left arm from shoulder to wrist, then use your left fist to thump your right arm. Use both fists to thump first one leg then the other from top to bottom. Finally, thump your torso from bottom to top. (Don't do this if you bruise easily due to blood-thinning medicine or for any other reason.)

▶ The stomach massage

If you have pain or discomfort in your gut try this after every meal. Place one hand on your stomach and the other hand on top. Now move them both together in a clockwise circular motion. Keep it up for at least two minutes.

▶ The eye massage

For eye strain, close your eyes and place the pads of your thumbs just under your eyebrows and just above the inner corners of your eyes. Making little circular movements gradually massage along your eyes just under your eyebrows. When you get to the outside corners, switch to your forefingers and work your way back underneath your eyes until you get back to your starting point. Repeat several times.

▶ The headache massage

For tension headaches, locate the little indentations in your temples close to the outermost points of your eyebrows. Using one or two fingers each side, massage this area with circular motions then gradually work your way along your forehead close to the hairline (or, if you're a man with receding hair, where your hairline used to be).

▶ The tennis ball self-massage

Here's an ingenious way of massaging the parts of your body you can't normally reach. All you need is a tennis ball. The idea is to trap it between the part of your body you want to massage and either the wall or the floor. It's not for a whole body massage but to deal with one or two problem areas.

Let's say, for example, you want to massage your lower back to the left of your spine. First warm the area with a hot water bottle or heat pad. Then stand with your back close to a wall, pop the ball into position and lean back against it. The pressure is right when it feels satisfying but not painful. Maintain the pressure for two to four minutes.

Try it now

If you have MSK pain and you happen to have a vibrator get it out and apply it where it hurts. A mains-powered model will be best.

Key idea

You don't have to be an expert to do good through massage. Even simple massage techniques increase blood flow, nourish cells, speed healing and boost production of the body's natural painkillers.

Heat and cold

We all like a hot bath when we're feeling a bit stiff and we're all familiar with a hot water bottle and the pleasure of lying in the sun. But is that all there is to it? Is it just all about comfort, like a child with a teddy?

In fact, our natural instinct to seek heat for aches and pains is well founded. One of the mechanisms is straightforward. Muscle strain creates a tension which, in turn, can reduce the blood supply and, therefore, the amount of oxygen reaching the cells, thus causing pain. Heat reverses that by dilating the blood vessels and restoring the blood supply. At the same time, the increased blood supply speeds recovery if there's any actual damage, and improves the flexibility of the soft tissues. As a bonus, the pleasant heat signals distract from the pain signals.

But, recently, scientists have demonstrated that there's something even more profound going on. Heat can actually deactivate pain at the molecular level in much the same way as painkilling tablets. If heat over 40°C is applied to the skin over the site of internal pain, heat receptors (known as TRPV1) are switched on, which in turn block pain receptors (known as P2X3) that cause the perception of pain. Research continues into a drug that will block P2X3, but in the meantime heat is a satisfactory method in many cases.

Dr Brian King at the Department of Physiology, University College London, who has led research into heat, in a speech to the Physiological Society, said that heat is also particularly effective for short-term pain relief for the body's hollow organs. 'The pain of colic, cystitis and period pain,' he explained, 'is caused by a temporary reduction in blood flow to or over-distension of hollow organs such as the bowel or uterus, causing local tissue damage and activating pain receptors.'

Remember this

In one study, researchers found heat was more effective at relieving lower back pain than either ibuprofen or paracetamol (acetaminophen).

There are various ways of applying heat:

▶ Hot water bottles. In the 16th century, metal bed warmers were filled with hot coals from the fire and used to warm the sheets before getting in. Quite soon someone had the idea of using containers of hot water which could safely be kept in the bed. Initially they were made of glass, earthenware, zinc, copper and even wood until the hot water bottle as we know it was invented by the Croatian engineer Slavoljub Penkala (1871–1922).

▶ Microwave heating pads. These contain a gel and can be heated in a microwave oven.

▶ Chemical pads. Hot water bottles and microwave pads are cumbersome. Chemical pads have the advantage that they can be stuck to the body and be invisible under clothes. Generally they contain reagents which, when the pad is squeezed hard enough, mix and create heat lasting eight to ten hours. Their disadvantage is that they're expensive and can be used only once. However, there are reusable versions containing a supersaturated solution of sodium acetate.

▶ Electric pads. These are mostly used by professional therapists. It would only be worth buying one for home use if you have a chronic condition.

▶ Infrared lamps. Good as surface heating can be, it's limited by the fact that the temperature of the heat device shouldn't exceed more than about 42°C, the heat being transferred from the surface of the skin to the lower levels by conduction. One method of getting the heat more directly where it's needed is to use infrared radiation. The sensation is very much like lying in the sun. Note that IR-B and IR-C rays have very little penetration – for a useful effect you need IR-A.

▶ Saunas and steam rooms. Most people's perception is that wet heat (as in a steam room) gets into the body faster. However, research by Regina M. Fink, clearly showed that dry heat (as in a sauna) was more effective at causing vasodilation, one of the key benefits of heat therapy. In one study published in Clinical Rheumatology, 17 patients with rheumatoid arthritis and 17 with ankylosing spondylitis, were given eight sessions in an infrared sauna over a four week period. (An infrared sauna uses infrared lamps rather than traditional heaters.) Reductions in pain, stiffness and fatigue were described as 'clinically significant' during the treatment. No adverse effects were reported.

Case study

'I practise quite a lot of sports and from time to time I get lower back pain. Sometimes it extends down my left leg. I used to take ibuprofen, which was quite effective, but then, somehow or other, I became allergic to it. Now I can't take any NSAIDs, which is an awful problem. Having a hot bath has always felt good so, next time I had back pain, I decided to see what would happen if I strapped a hot water bottle to my back. I held it in place using one of those corset-like back supports. I kept it there all afternoon and evening, refilling the bottle every hour. I was also able to wear it for a couple of hours in bed, because I always sleep on my side. When I woke up in the morning I was fine. No back pain and no stiffness. Great! Now, as soon as I feel the slightest hint of back trouble I get out the hot water bottle.' Peter (44)

Try it now

If you have an ache or pain right now, dig out the hot water bottle and see what it can do for you. You may need to experiment because the place that hurts may not be where the problem lies. Heat applied to the upper back and neck, for example, helps many people with tension headaches.

HEAT AND LABOUR PAINS

Can heat be used to reduce labour pains? It can if you opt for a water birth. The idea is that the water should be about the same temperature as the human body so the emerging baby remains in a fairly constant environment. It has nothing to do with pain reduction but it seems that, coincidentally, what suits the baby is also just high enough to have a significant impact on the mother's pain (35–37°C during the first stage of labour and 37–37.5°C in the second stage).

Verena Geissbühler and Jakob Eberhard at the Clinic for Obstetrics and Gynaecology in Frauenfeld, Switzerland, studied 7,508 births between 1991 and 1997, of which 2,014 were water births. They concluded that: 'Fewer painkillers are used in water births and the experience of birth itself is more satisfying…' Of the women who gave birth in (warm) water, nearly three-quarters (70.6 per cent) needed no painkillers, compared with 66.1 per cent of women using a Maia-birthing stool. Of those women who gave birth in bed, almost half (45.9 per cent) did need painkillers. Equally significant were the kinds of analgesics used. Women using water births mostly relied upon homeopathic remedies. More than a fifth of all women giving birth in water chose them and only 0.4 per cent were given the much more powerful epidural analgesics. By contrast, two per cent of women using the Maia-birthing stool were given epidurals and in the case of bed births the figure was eight per cent.

COLD

If heat is good, how come some people use ice when they have an injury? Good question. In 2010, a team of researchers led by Professor Lan Zhou at the Neuroinflammation Research Centre at the Cleveland Clinic in Ohio concluded that icing injuries to reduce inflammation actually *slows* healing. They found that inflamed cells produce large quantities of a hormone called insulin-like growth factor-1 (IGF-1) which significantly increases the rate of muscle regeneration. Using ice, then, looks like a mistake. And, indeed, it's been known for a long time that excess anti-inflammatory medicine such as cortisone slows wound healing.

So is ice never of any use? It seems to be a matter of timing and degree. The consensus is that ice is helpful during the acute stage (say up to 48 or even 72 hours after the injury). Leave it in place for no more than 20 minutes and wait 40 minutes before using it again. Heat at this stage will increase bleeding, swelling and pain. But once the inflammation has begun to subside, heat will relieve muscle tightness, ease joints and reduce pain.

If you're engaged in some kind of sporting activity over several days, icing can also help to keep you going. The problem then is Delayed Onset Muscle Soreness (DOMS). DOMS is what you get the day after a really gruelling day of exercise. According to a study published in the International Journal of Sports Medicine in 2008, ice baths may aid recovery. The ideal temperature seems to be around 10°–15°C for about 10 minutes. Most people would probably prefer the DOMS.

Key idea

* Use cold after exercise or physical strain to reduce inflammation
* Use heat when you get up to relax muscles and joints
* At bedtime use heat again.

Remember this

If you've twisted your foot running, or something like that, and the area is swollen, remember the acronym RICE. It stands for Rest, Ice, Compression, Elevation. In other words, ice the area as described above, apply a compression bandage and use a stool or cushions to keep the part up and immobile. But switch to heat after two or three days.

Acupuncture

Although acupuncture remains controversial, the weight of scientific evidence is now more for it than against. At the time of writing, the National Institute for Health and Clinical Excellence (NICE) in the UK only sees acupuncture as useful for lower back pain, chronic tension-type headache and migraine. However, the World Health Organization (WHO) says acupuncture is effective for treating 28 conditions, an impressive endorsement.

Specifically as regards pain, a 2007 a study published in the American *Archives of Internal Medicine* found that, over six months, acupuncture was more effective at treating lower back pain than medication, exercise and physical therapy. A 2009 review by the Cochrane Collaboration (an independent, international non-profit organization) found that acupuncture was more effective than routine care for migraines and with fewer adverse effects than preventative drugs. A 2011 analysis of eight Cochrane reviews concluded that acupuncture is effective in the treatment of migraines, neck disorders, tension headaches and peripheral joint osteoarthritis.

Most persuasive of all, in 2012 researchers analysed the results from 29 high quality trials involving nearly 18,000 patients with chronic pain in the UK, Germany and the USA. All were receiving conventional treatment. According to lead author, Dr Andrew Vickers, the average pain level reported by patients prior to acupuncture was 60/100. As soon as they were told they were entering an acupuncture trial – and this is particularly interesting – the average pain level fell to 43. This is a well-known effect of trials. So what did the acupuncture add? Those who received 'sham' acupuncture, in which needles were inserted at random, reported pain levels of 35. Those who had genuine acupuncture, with needles carefully placed in accordance with the theory of meridians, rated their pain at an average of 30.

From this huge study it's very clear that the placebo effect plays a role. But it also seems that something more is going on. The needling obviously made a significant contribution. On the other hand, the difference between random needling and the needling of acupuncture points was not huge. And that's been the finding of many studies. The 2009 Cochrane review mentioned above not only found that acupuncture worked, it also found that 'sham acupuncture' worked just as well. In the 'Vickers' analysis it's quite possible the medical staff giving the 'sham' acupuncture just did not convey the same feeling of reassurance and competence as when needles were placed in specific points. That may have been enough to account for the fairly small difference between genuine and sham acupuncture, in which case the traditional theory of acupuncture falls apart. But what is undeniable is that placing the needles into the body, whether in special places or just at random, does something useful.

HOW ACUPUNCTURE WORKS

James Reston, who worked for the New York Times, received acupuncture in China in 1971 for post-operative pain. In a subsequent article he described how the acupuncturist 'inserted three long, thin needles into the outer part of my right elbow and below my knees and manipulated them.' The immediate effect was to send 'ripples of pain' racing through his limbs. The full treatment took about 20 minutes after which, Reston reported, 'there was a noticeable relaxation of the pressure and distension within an hour and no recurrence of the problem thereafter.' The article provoked enormous interest in America and did a great deal to promote acupuncture there.

I've interviewed several people who, like Reston, were cured in a single session. But more typically acupuncture involves about a dozen weekly or fortnightly sessions of 30 minutes each. While you're lying down, the acupuncturist will insert single use, disposable, sterile needles so fine that initially there will be no pain. However, once the needles have reached the target depth there should be a deep aching sensation. Generally, that would be around a quarter of an inch to an inch (6 mm – 25 mm) but in the buttocks, for example, it could be as deep as three to four inches (75 mm – 100 mm). The needles may be manipulated in some way or they may simply be left in place for about 20 minutes.

The traditional Chinese theory is that 'life energy' known as chi or qi or gi flows through meridians in the body. Illness results when this life force is blocked or disturbed. Acupuncture points (tsubos) are like manholes, giving access to these energy pathways, and the needles are the tools by which normal flow can be restored.

Western science, it has to be said, has never been able to find any evidence for such meridians. If they don't exist, how would acupuncture achieve more than a placebo effect? The most obvious answer is by provoking the release of endorphins, the body's own natural painkillers. In 2010, a study on mice led by Dr Maiken Nedergaard discovered that acupuncture also releases adenosine, another natural painkiller. After 30-minute acupuncture sessions, the level of adenosine close to the needles was 24 times higher than normal.

IS ACUPUNCTURE DANGEROUS?

A study published in September 2012 revealed that in a three-year period in the UK where acupuncture was given on the National Health there were five cases of punctured lungs, 63 cases in which patients lost consciousness, and 59 cases in which the acupuncturist forgot to remove one or more needles at the end of treatment. Unfortunately there were no figures on the total use of acupuncture by the NHS over the three years but other studies have put the frequency of 'mild adverse incidents' for all acupuncturists in the UK at between approximately 7 per cent and 15 per cent, so acupuncture is not without some risk.

Remember this

When needles are being pushed deep into the body it's vitally important to find an experienced acupuncture specialist. Before submitting to the needles, try to get personal recommendations and check out the person's level of experience very carefully. In the UK, your acupuncturist should be registered with a recognized body such as the British Acupuncture Council (BacC) or the British Medical Acupuncture Society. In the USA most states require a practitioner to hold a Master of Acupuncture & Oriental Medicine degree or equivalent from an institution accepted by the Accreditation Commission for Acupuncture and Oriental Medicine (ACAOM).

Case study

'I urgently had to drive from Amsterdam to the south of France when I had severe back pain. It made it difficult to sit for any length of time or to apply foot pressure to the clutch. So I decided to try acupuncture. Shortly after the needles went in I began to feel strange. My girlfriend was watching me and said I had turned green. I had the sensation almost as if poisons were being driven out of me. After the session I stood up and the pain was gone. Next day I drove all the way to Perpignan without a problem. The day after that I had some discomfort but nothing like the pain I had originally experienced.' Guy (40)

Shiatsu and acupressure

Some practitioners use the terms 'shiatsu' and 'acupressure' interchangeably, while others consider shiatsu as embracing a wider range of techniques. For simplicity, I'll use the term 'shiatsu'. The essence is that, rather than using needles, pressure is applied to the tsubos mostly using fingers but also occasionally hands, the elbow or a special device.

As opposed to acupuncture, very little scientific research has been conducted into shiatsu performed by a therapist. But there has been research into the most well-known of the shiatsu devices, which is the wristband that presses on the P6 tsubo. In one study in the coronary care unit at Torbay Hospital, Devon, England, patients who had suffered myocardial infarction were less likely to experience nausea and vomiting 4 to 20 hours later if they had wristbands. Only 18 per cent with P6 wristbands experienced nausea or vomiting during that period, compared with 32 per cent receiving placebo acupressure and 43 per cent who had neither. All three groups also received standard antiemetic drug therapy. However, a study of 700 cancer patients at the University of Rochester Medical Center, came to the conclusion that only those who expected the wristbands to work experienced any benefit.

So the evidence is inconclusive but, in fact, a wristband is not able to exert the same kind of pressure that a therapist would. I have interviewed people who are convinced shiatsu helped them and the case study below is my own. The best advice is to try a bona fide shiatsu therapist who practises a wide range of techniques, including massage, and see if it works for you. In the UK, be sure to check that the therapist is an Acupressure Member of the Acupuncture Society (MAcSAp) or similar. In the USA, look for certification as an Asian Bodywork Therapist (ABT).

Try it now

One of the most famous tsubos in acupressure is the so-called HeGu (also known as Go Koku, Meeting Mountains, or Large Intestine 4). Here's what you do when you have a headache or dental pain. While looking at the back of your left hand, press the side of your thumb against your forefinger. As the muscle swells up, note the highest point. Now spread your thumb and forefinger and place the thumb of your other (right) hand where the high point was. That's HeGu. Using the forefinger of your right hand for support, press the tip and nail of your right thumb into HeGu. Some practitioners recommend pressing three times for fifteen seconds each time, others say it may be necessary to hold it for several minutes. (Note that if you're left-handed you may find it easier to use the tsubo in your right hand.) Does it work? Try it and see.

The placebo effect

You may imagine the placebo effect is the equivalent of saying the problem was 'all in the mind'. That there was nothing really wrong in the first place. If you did think that then you're in for a shock. The truth is astonishing.

Every successful treatment includes a substantial placebo effect.

In other words, if you're in pain and are given some kind of treatment which makes you feel better, part of that success will be due to the placebo effect. We know this from numerous studies.

But that's not the end of the incredible story of the placebo. The psychologist Frederick Evans, a distinguished researcher into hypnosis, discovered something even more amazing. In his book *Placebo: Theory, Research and Mechanism* he explained it like this: 'The effectiveness of the placebo is proportional to the apparent effectiveness of the active analgesic agent.'

For analgesics he put the role of the placebo at 56 per cent. In other words, if you were to be given a weak painkiller such as aspirin, 56 per cent of the benefit would be down to the placebo effect. And if you were given a relatively strong painkiller such as morphine, it would still be the case that 56 per cent of the effect would be due to the placebo response. In other words, the more powerful the treatment, the more powerful the placebo response.

He found this phenomenon worked for other types of drug as well. For sleeping pills he put the placebo effect at 58 per cent, and for tricyclic antidepressants at 59 per cent.

Of course, nothing can make the body act in a way in which it's not capable. No amount of placebo can make a human body regenerate a lost limb, for example. But, according to Ernest Rossi Ph.D., who has made a detailed study of such phenomena, the placebo effect is especially powerful in problems involving the autonomic nervous system, the endocrine system, or the immune system, such as:

▶ Asthma

▶ Colds and flu

▶ Diabetes

▶ Headaches

▶ Hypertension

▶ Menstrual Pain

▶ Multiple sclerosis

▶ Rheumatoid arthritis

▶ Ulcers

▶ Warts.

Key idea

When something is said to work entirely or partly through a placebo effect it tends to be dismissed as a useful therapy. However, that's not at all logical. If something works, it works. As Norman Cousins, author of *Anatomy of an Illness* wrote: 'The placebo is the doctor who resides within.'

The extreme opposite of the placebo is the nocebo (from the Latin meaning 'I will harm'). A nocebo is something that causes a person to feel ill or become ill, even though it's completely harmless, due to pessimism and fear. The interesting thing is that nocebo pain is just as real as any other pain. In February 2011 a team led by Oxford professor Irene Tracey showed that when volunteers felt nocebo pain an MRI scanner showed there was corresponding 'pain activity' in the brain. Another team, led by Fabrizio Benedetti at the University of Turin, has uncovered one of the neurochemicals responsible for nocebo pain. It's called cholecystokinin and when it's blocked by a drug patients feel no nocebo pain.

So it's clear that mental attitudes have a great deal to do with not only the sensation of pain but also with recovery from illness. In extreme cases, people die from fear. Walter Cannon MD (1871–1945) was a pioneer in the investigation of what he called 'voodoo death'. It was he who coined the phrase 'flight or fight'. He also refined ideas about homeostasis or the way the body maintains a fairly constant state. Cannon described cases in which men and women who had been 'cursed' or had accidentally broken a serious taboo, immediately fell ill and died within hours or days. Some have questioned the accuracy of his accounts and his explanation of the mechanisms involved has now been superseded. But there's plenty of evidence that people can die of fear and hopelessness, and not just in pre-technological societies. In 1992 the Southern Medical Journal reported the case of a man who died not long after being told he had liver cancer. The autopsy, however, showed the tumour had not progressed and should not have been fatal, suggesting the man actually died of fear.

How? It seems that in response to a massive stress, hormones are secreted from the brain, adrenal and pituitary glands that cause cardiac arrhythmias, weakness, vascular collapse and, ultimately, death.

Key idea

In a Swedish study in 2012 it was found that even when stimuli were presented outside of conscious awareness pain could be reduced or increased by placebo and nocebo effects. In other words, you don't even have to be consciously aware of a placebo for it to act on you.

Remember this

Let me now try to engender a little of the placebo effect if you're suffering from cancer. According to the American Cancer Society, the five-year relative survival rate for all cancers diagnosed between 1975 and 1977 was 49 per cent. For those diagnosed between 2001 and 2007 it was 67 per cent, a significant improvement. (Relative survival compares survival among cancer patients to that of people not diagnosed with cancer who are of the same age, race and gender.) Even since 2007, treatments have improved yet again. So it can be said that if you've been diagnosed recently then your chances of surviving at least five years are extremely good.

Focus points

* Massage has been proven to be a successful treatment for pain from various sources
* With a little ingenuity it's quite possible to give yourself an effective massage
* Heat can be as effective as ibuprofen in some circumstances
* The weight of evidence is more for acupuncture than against it, although it may not work in the way traditionalists believe
* Every successful treatment, of whatever kind, always includes a placebo effect.

Next step

Massage, heat and acupuncture are essentially passive treatments. In the next chapter we'll be coming at things from a very different angle. We'll be seeing how something far more active can unleash the body's own natural painkillers.

Exercise therapy

In this chapter you will learn:

- ▶ *how endorphins, the body's own natural painkillers, increase with exercise*
- ▶ *how correct posture can cure MSK pain*
- ▶ *how to exercise for maximum painkilling effect.*

A lot of times when you play ... you get this adrenaline that blocks pain.

Venus Williams, five times Wimbledon champion

When people are actually in pain they tend to avoid exercise. And, of course, for some people exercise is impossible. But for those who *can* exercise, Venus Williams is right. Exercise reduces pain, although adrenaline is only one of the chemicals involved and tends to be short-lived. But exercise is much more than a short-term painkiller. Several studies have convincingly proved that people who exercise have significantly less sensitivity to pain *in the long term* than people who don't exercise. The explanation lies in endorphins.

Endorphins are the body's own natural painkillers. The word is a combination of 'endogenous' (meaning 'made in the body') and morphine. In other words, the body can actually make a substance akin to the powerful analgesic derived from the opium poppy. And one way of getting the body to produce endorphins is to exercise vigorously. A six-mile run stimulates endorphins equivalent to 10 mg of morphine – roughly a standard painkilling dose.

There are other aspects to exercise, too. Think of a stiff, rusty hinge. 'Rest' it and eventually it will lock solid. But work it gently every day by opening and closing it and it will remain functional. Then think of the load on the hinge. A door that weighs 225 pounds will wear it out much sooner than a door that weighs 150 pounds. That's to say, exercise helps to keep you supple and control your weight thus limiting the strain on your spine and joints.

So let's assess where you are now.

Diagnostic test

The first five questions are designed to check your attitude to exercise – in each group choose the answer that most closely represents you. The final five questions are designed to make an assessment of your 'anti-pain fitness'.

1 The thought of exercise:

   a Fills me with optimism
   b Bores me
   c Terrifies me.

2 When I exercise I feel:

   a Happy and exhilarated
   b Okay
   c Tired and miserable.

3 I exercise:

   a Vigorously for at least twenty minutes three times a week – or more
   b A bit at weekends
   c By doing the gardening, the chores and the shopping – that's enough exercise for anyone.

4 Exercise:

   a Reduces my pain
   b Has no discernible effect on my pain
   c Makes my pain worse.

5 Exercise:

   a Increases the mobility of my joints and keeps me supple
   b Has no beneficial effects
   c Makes my joints worse and increases stiffness.

6 My Body Mass Index (BMI)* is:

   a 20–23
   b 24
   c 25–27, or under 20
   d Over 27.

*To calculate BMI see the explanation at the end of the questionnaire.

7 My resting heart rate (my pulse when I wake up in the morning and before I get out of bed) is:

   a Under 50
   b 50–60
   c 60–70
   d 70–80

e 80–90

f Over 90.

8 After warming up and with my legs straight I can touch:

   a The floor with the palms of my hands
   b The floor with the tips of my fingers
   c My ankle bones
   d My calves.

9 In one minute I can do the following number of sit-ups:

   a More than 50
   b 40–50
   c 30–40
   d 20–30
   e 10–20.

(Don't do this if you have a back problem. To do sit-ups, lie on your back on the carpet, knees bent, heels about 45 cm (18 inches) from your buttocks, feet flat on the floor shoulder-width apart and anchored under a heavy piece of furniture. Then sit up. Your hands should be on the sides of your head. When reclining you only need to touch your shoulders to the floor. If you can't do sit-ups but can do crunches, do them instead. Begin a crunch as for a sit-up but keep your lower back on the floor and raise only your head and shoulders.)

10 I can walk half a mile in:

   a Under 6 minutes
   b 6–7 minutes
   c 7–8 minutes
   d 8–9 minutes
   e 9–10 minutes
   f Over 10 minutes.

(Measure the distance along a flat stretch of road/pavement using your car.)

▶ **Your score**

As regards questions one to five:

▶ If you mostly answered 'a' you obviously have a very positive attitude towards exercise and, hopefully, are already gaining some benefit from that. You should find exercise therapy fairly easy.

▶ If you mostly answered 'b' you're less than enthusiastic about exercise and you're also highly sceptical about its painkilling potential but, hopefully, you'll be willing to give it a go.

▶ If you answered mostly 'c' you're probably now bristling with indignation at the very suggestion that exercise could help your pain. If that's the case, try to keep an open mind and stop thinking of exercise as either a chore or an irrelevance. There are all kinds of fun ways of going about it, as you'll discover later in the chapter.

As regards question six:

▶ A BMI of 24 is considered the cut-off between being a healthy weight and being overweight. The higher you are over 24 the more you're subjecting your joints to potentially painful stresses. So 20–23 would be really good and 24 is okay. But anything over 24 risks being unhealthy (as does anything under 20, although for different reasons).

*Here's how to do the BMI calculation:

Step 1. Get hold of a calculator.

Step 2. Work out the square of your height in metres (that is, your height in metres multiplied by itself – see example).

Step 3. Divide your weight in kilograms by the number you obtained in Step 2.

Example:

Suppose you weigh 58 kilos and are 1.6 metres tall. The square of 1.6 (1.6×1.6) is 2.56. So your BMI is 58 divided by 2.56, which is 22.6.

If you only know your weight in pounds, you can convert it to kilograms by dividing the number of pounds by 2.2; to convert inches to metres, divide the number of inches by 39.37.

As regards questions seven to ten:

► Calculate your individual scores according to the following tables and then add the four numbers together to obtain your 'anti-pain fitness' score.

Question 7

	Men	Women
a	23	25
b	18	20
c	13	15
d	8	10
e	3	5
f	0	0

Question 8

	Men			Women		
	Under 30	30-50	Over 50	Under 30	30-50	Over 50
a	15	20	25	13	18	23
b	10	15	20	8	13	18
c	8	13	18	6	11	16
d	5	10	15	3	8	13

Question 9

	Men			Women		
	Under 30	30-50	Over 50	Under 30	30–50	Over 50
a	20	25	–	25	–	–
b	15	20	25	20	25	–
c	10	15	20	15	20	25
d	5	10	15	10	15	20
e	2	5	10	5	10	15

Question 10

	Men			Women		
	Under 30	30-50	Over 50	Under 30	30–50	Over 50
a	20	25	–	25	–	–
b	15	20	25	20	25	–
c	10	15	20	15	20	25
d	5	10	15	10	15	20
e	1	5	10	5	10	15
f	–	–	–	–	–	–

What your 'anti-pain fitness' score means (questions 7 to 10):

▶ If you scored 65 or over you must be an athlete of some sort and should be enjoying the pain relief produced by all those endorphins, but you're possibly inflicting some pain on yourself, too – don't overdo it.

▶ If you scored 45 to 64 you're in pretty good shape. Just keep on with the exercise regime that you're already following.

▶ If you scored 20 to 44 you could gain a tremendous amount by exercising more vigorously and more often. In a way you're very lucky because you're going to improve rapidly once you start exercising regularly – you'll notice a difference in pain relief and mood very quickly.

▶ If you scored 19 or less it may well be that a lack of physical fitness is playing a significant role in your pain. But don't fling yourself immediately into anything too strenuous. You're obviously not used to exercise and, for various reasons, you may not have many exercise options open to you. Consult your doctor to work out a suitable programme and see the notes on 'pacing' below.

Pacing

If your pain and state of health don't permit vigorous movement you should nevertheless be aiming to do something and, over time, to increase your activity to the level at which you can generate those painkilling endorphins. The way to achieve that is through 'pacing'.

Pacing is a method of increasing physical activity without increasing your pain. Pacing means stopping an activity *before* it becomes too painful, not *when* it becomes too painful. It means curtailing activities today so as to avoid painful repercussions tomorrow. Always be guided by your pain and never overdo things.

The idea is to work out your current activity level or 'baseline' and then to increase it very gradually. Here's how.

▶ Day 1: Think of how much of an activity you can comfortably manage. Let's say five minutes of walking. Try it out and make a note of how many minutes you actually did achieve.

▶ Day 2: Taking into account how much you managed on Day 1, set a new target (higher or lower) and try it out. Make a note of what you actually achieved.

▶ Day 3: Taking into account how much you managed on Day 2, set a new target (higher or lower) and try it out. Again make a note of what you actually achieved. Work out the average of the first three days by adding together the three 'scores' and dividing by three. Your baseline is 80 per cent (four-fifths) of that figure.

Now that you have your baseline you can work out a programme for increasing your level of activity. Initially, aim for something like a 10 per cent increase after every two days. For example, if your baseline is 5 minutes of walking then you should aim for 5 minutes and 30 seconds on days three and four, 6 minutes on days five and six, and so on. After three weeks recalculate your baseline and set new targets. It's not always a case of increasing the time spent on an activity. Depending on what it is, you could also increase the speed, or the amount of weight, or the number of repetitions. You can apply this principal to all kinds of activities, from housework or mowing the lawn to swimming or weight lifting.

As you reach higher levels of activity you may find that 10 per cent increases after every two days are too tiring or simply impossible. In that case, aim for 10 per cent after every week, or even 5 per cent. A constant increase is the aim, however small. The key point is that you should never do so much that you have to cut back the following day.

Remember this

It's essential to keep a diary of your activity so you'll know what progress you're making and so that you can reset your baseline from time to time.

Simple 'anti-pain' exercises

Let's kick off with some easy exercises that you should aim to do every day if you're physically able. They're designed to increase strength and mobility and reduce MSK pain.

EXERCISES TO SUPPORT THE BACK

If you regularly have lower back pain you should be able to reduce flare ups by strengthening some of the muscles that support your back – the abdominals (the muscles you tense to hold your stomach in). When your abdominals are strong so you reduce the strain on your back when, for example, you bend down and lift something heavy. But how can you strengthen your abs without hurting your back even more? Here are two exercises that will do the trick. The first one is the crunch.

1 Lie on your back with your knees bent, feet flat on the floor, and your hands behind your head.

2 Inhaling, and with your abs braced, raise your shoulders and head slightly from the floor. Don't use your arms to pull your head up.

3 Keeping your shoulders and head off the floor, breathe normally for 10 seconds.

4 Exhaling, lower your shoulders and head to the floor.

5 Repeat five times.

The hanging straight-leg raise is a more powerful exercise but you will need a bar of some kind that you can hang from.

1 With your legs very slightly bent, raise them slowly in front of you to the horizontal position.

2 Very slowly lower your legs down again.

3 Repeat as many times as you can.

HIP ROTATION

This exercise is designed to increase the flexibility of your hips.

1 Lie on your back with your knees bent, your feet flat on the floor, your arms stretched out sideways and the palms of your hands downwards.

2 Cross your left leg over your right and allow both of them together to topple sideways (to the left).

3 Hold the position for 10 seconds.

4 Repeat five times on each side.

CROSS-LEG STRETCH

This exercise is designed to improve the mobility of your lower back and hips.

1 Stand with your legs well apart and your arms stretched up above your head.

2 Keeping your legs straight, bend gently forward from the waist and try to touch your left foot with your right hand; if you can't touch your foot touch your ankle. Hold the position for two seconds.

3 Straighten up and repeat on the other side, touching your right foot or ankle with your left hand and holding the position for two seconds.

4 Repeat on both sides a total of five times.

TREE POSE

This is a famous pose for improving balance.

1 Stand with your feet together and arms by your sides.

2 Lift your right leg and place the sole of your right foot against the inside of your left knee.

3 Inhaling, slowly raise your arms above your head.

4 Endeavour to hold the pose for ten seconds, breathing normally.

5 Exhaling, lower your arms and put your foot back on the floor.

6 Repeat the procedure, but this time placing the left foot against the right knee.

7 Repeat the whole thing on both sides three more times.

THE HALF SPINAL TWIST

This is an exercise to increase the mobility of the hip, knee and spine.

1 Kneel down with your legs together and sit back on your feet.

2 Move your buttocks off your feet to the right so that you're sitting on the floor beside your feet.

3 Lift your left leg over your right and place your left foot on the floor beside your right knee; meanwhile your right heel should remain close to your buttocks.

4 Keeping your back straight, stretch your arms out to the sides and twist around to the left.

5 Bring your right arm down on the *outside* of the left knee and take hold of your left foot in your right hand. This should be quite difficult.

6 Place your left hand on the floor behind you.

7 Exhaling, twist as far as possible to the left, looking over your left shoulder.

8 Repeat the whole sequence to the other side.

Remember this

You're probably familiar with the phrase, 'use it or lose it'. How very true. Your body doesn't like to waste resources maintaining things that might never be used. If you spend most of the day sitting down in front of a computer screen your body will conclude that it needn't waste time building you a nice set of abdominal muscles. On the other hand, it might produce lots of tight collagen to hold you in your customary position. That's not good.

Never spend more than an hour at a time sitting in front of your screen – or anything else. Get up, walk around a bit, and do the following before resuming work:

1 Put your arms straight out behind your back and clasp your hands together with your fingers interlaced.

2 Bring your shoulder blades towards one another and down.

3 Tilt your head back a bit.

4 Hold for a few seconds, release, and repeat twice more.

This should help your neck and, consequently, deter back aches and headaches.

The Alexander technique

We have to thank an obliging horse for the Alexander technique. Frederick Matthias Alexander was a Shakespearian orator in Australia who suffered voice loss. Doctors could do nothing for him so he developed his own treatment which involved relearning how to stand, move and breathe. His technique would probably never have become widely known had he not won £750 on a horse race and bought a boat ticket to England.

Essentially Alexander believed that all kinds of pains, not just voice problems, were due to uneven distribution of weight and poor posture over many years. One way of describing Alexander technique is to say it's a way of learning to get rid of harmful tensions in your body. It's moving mindfully, with ease, freedom and balance.

Does it work?

A team headed by Paul Little, a Professor of Primary Care Research at Southampton University, followed a total of 579 people who had been suffering back pain for three or more weeks and who scored above four on the Roland disability scale. (The scale is reproduced below if you would like to know your own score.) Having been assessed, the subjects were randomly assigned to one of eight treatment groups. One of the groups included six Alexander technique lessons, while another included 24. The subjects were then reassessed after three months and again after one year and compared with controls.

The conclusion was that the 24 Alexander technique lessons provided the most effective strategy out of the various treatments and that just six lessons combined with exercise were 72 per cent as effective.

Following on from that study, Dr Stuart McClean of University of the West of England, Bristol, led an enquiry into the practicality of offering Alexander technique to outpatients at the Pain Clinic at St Michael's Hospital, Bristol. He and his team followed 43 patients with chronic or recurrent pain. Three-quarters of the patients had back pain and none of the 43 was getting better with conventional treatment. The 43 received instruction in Alexander technique in 2010 and 2011. Each patient received six weekly one-to-one sessions. The result was a substantial reduction in the use of pain medication (and a significant saving in other NHS costs as well).

In the UK, the National Institute for Health and Clinical Excellence (NICE) recommends exercise along with acupuncture and manual therapy as suitable treatments for persistent non-specific low back pain. The Alexander technique is included in the exercise category and you should be able to obtain it on the National Health.

During lessons, which usually last 30 to 45 minutes, your teacher will observe your current posture and your way of moving and guide you into the correct forms. Around 20 lessons are usually recommended but it's apparent from the research quoted above that just six lessons can make a substantial difference.

Key idea

Lessons in Alexander technique are expensive because, whether in a group or individual setting, they involve a lot of one-on-one time. Pilates is a cheaper alternative which may well prove just as effective in your particular case.

▶ The Roland disability scale for back pain

Put a tick by each item that describes your situation. Your score is the number of ticks. When you go to see your doctor or other professionals let them know your score.

1 I stay at home most of the time because of my back

2 I change position frequently to try to get my back comfortable

3 I walk more slowly than usual because of my back

4 Because of my back I am not doing any of the jobs that I usually do around the house

5 Because of my back, I use a handrail to get upstairs

6 Because of my back, I lie down to rest more often

7 Because of my back, I have to hold on to something to get out of an easy chair

8 Because of my back, I try to get other people to do things for me

9 I get dressed more slowly than usual because of my back

10 I only stand for short periods of time because of my back

11 Because of my back, I try not to bend or kneel down

12 I find it difficult to get out of a chair because of my back

13 My back is painful almost all the time

14 I find it difficult to turn over in bed because of my back

15 My appetite is not very good because of my back pain

16 I have trouble putting on my socks (or stockings) because of the pain in my back

17 I only walk short distances because of my back

18 I sleep less well because of my back

19 Because of my back pain, I get dressed with help from someone else

20 I sit down for most of the day because of my back

21 I avoid heavy jobs around the house because of my back

22 Because of my back pain, I am more irritable and bad tempered with people than usual

23 Because of my back, I go upstairs more slowly than usual

24 I stay in bed most of the time because of my back.

More vigorous exercise

A little exercise is good, more is better. In this section we'll be looking at the way vigorous exercise unleashes the body's own natural painkillers. But first, a word of caution.

▶ **Warning**

If you haven't been exercising regularly and have any of the following characteristics you should check with your doctor before beginning an exercise regime:

* over 35 and a smoker
* over 40 and inactive
* diabetic
* at risk of heart disease
* high blood pressure
* high cholesterol
* experience chest pains while exercising
* difficulty breathing during mild exertion.

Remember this

Exercise should not be painful. If you feel pain in a new place, or additional pain in an existing place, you're doing too much, or doing it in the wrong way.

HOW EXERCISE COMBATS PAIN

When you think about it, it's not hard to understand how humans evolved in such a way that exercise would reduce pain. Our ancestors had to be capable of vigorous activity if they were to eat. When their muscles screamed for respite, those whose bodies produced chemicals to ease the pain were the ones who ran down the prey and got the food. Logically, they were also the ones evolution selected. Well, that's a simplistic way of putting it but right in essence. Nowadays we only have to be capable of lifting a can off a shelf but our bodies remain unchanged. So if we want to benefit from those same chemicals we have to make a deliberate effort to exercise. Here are some of the chemicals:

▶ Endorphins. We've already met these morphine-like substances. In addition to combating pain they also promote happiness and are one of the ingredients in the 'runner's high'.

▶ Phenylethylamine (PEA). This chemical is a powerful antidepressant according to researchers at Rush University and the Center for Creative Development, Chicago. Scientists at Nottingham Trent University in the UK have shown that PEA levels increase significantly following exercise. It's also found in chocolate as well as some fizzy drinks but the absorption appears to be minimal. Oh yes, you can also generate PEA by falling in love.

▶ Noradrenaline/norepinephrine (NE). When generated by exercise, noradrenaline tends to make you feel happy, confident, positive and expansive.

▶ Serotonin. The link with exercise isn't so strong for this one but serotonin is a neurotransmitter for happiness and there's reason to think exercise elevates its level in the brain.

In addition, moderate exercise lowers the level of:

▶ Cortisol. Also known as hydrocortisone, cortisol is a hormone that increases in response to stress. In the short term it reduces pain sensitivity, which is helpful in an accident, but chronically high cortisol levels decrease bone formation, leading to osteoporosis, may cause loss of collagen (the main component of connective tissue), depress the immune system, and increase gastric acid secretion (which is why stress often leads to heartburn and pain from ulcers).

But those chemicals are not the whole story. Blood supply is another major factor. As we saw in Chapter 5, blocked blood vessels reduce the supply of oxygen and nutrients to tissues, causing both acute and chronic pain. A healthier diet is certainly one part of the answer. Exercise is another.

There's plenty of evidence for this. Common age-related changes to the endothelium (a protective layer of cells inside the blood vessels) increase the likelihood of atherosclerosis (hardening) and thrombosis, leading to restricted blood flow and, potentially, to strokes and heart attacks. But those changes are not inevitable. Researchers led by Dr Stefano Taddei studied elderly men and women (average age 66) who exercised regularly and found that they had blood vessels that functioned as well as those of young adults (average age 27).

And it's never too late. In a randomized controlled trial involving subjects with pre-existing coronary artery disease, Dr Dean Ornish, Clinical Professor of Medicine at the University of California, demonstrated it was actually possible to *reverse* atherosclerosis by giving up smoking, following a plant-based diet, using stress reduction techniques and, crucially, practising moderate exercise.

In a study specifically into low back pain (Vijay B. Vad, A. L. Bhat, and Y. Tarabichi), sufferers were divided into two groups. One group was allowed the painkiller hydrocodone as necessary and wore a cryobrace (a support that also cools the tissues) for 15 minutes before going to bed. The other group did the same but in addition exercised for 15 minutes three times a week. After one year:

▶ 70 per cent of the exercise group, compared with only 33 per cent of the non-exercise group, reported better than 50 per cent pain reduction.

▶ The exercise group took less time off work than the non-exercise group.

▶ The exercise group had less symptom recurrence than the non-exercise group.

▶ The exercise group took fewer hydrocodone tablets than the non-exercise group (except during the first three weeks).

Remember, those very positive results were achieved with only 45 minutes of exercise per week. That's not very much. With more exercise the improvement should be even more dramatic.

And there's another bonus, too. It transpires that exercise also protects the brain. A team of researchers at the University of North Carolina compared the brain scans of a dozen volunteers aged 60 to 76, six of whom had been exercising for at least three hours a week over the previous 10 years, and six of whom had exercised less than one hour a week. The exercise group had better cerebral blood flow as well as more small blood vessels in the brain. It's thought that improved blood supply means better brain function. In addition, it seems that regular exercise produces an immune messenger in the brain called interleukin-6 which protects against inflammatory damage. In another twist, repetitive physical activities such as jogging 'shut down' the left side of the brain (logical thought), freeing up the right brain (creative thought). It's a kind of meditation and it's why solutions to seemingly intractable problems often appear 'by magic' when exercising.

Finally, there's the issue of thermogenics. Exercise increases the body's core temperature, which in turn relaxes muscles, which in turn reduces pain and induces a feeling of tranquillity.

Case study

'I work as a farrier. That's really tough on the back. Yet, unlike many people with jobs far less physically demanding, I seldom suffer from back problems. I certainly never get back pain during the working week. If I get the aches it's usually on a Sunday after I've been taking it easy over the weekend. The worst time for backache is if I go on holiday and just lie on the beach. By working I keep my back pain free.' Jack (27)

Key idea

If the word 'exercise' bothers you, call it something else. For example, you could call it, 'enjoying your body', or 'revelling in sensuality' or 'optimizing your physicality'. Birds swoop. Lambs gambol. Horses canter. Dolphins leap. Why? For the sheer pleasure of having a body and the thrill of moving it. Better still, why not call it 'my pain medicine'.

How exercise combats pain-related depression

Chronic pain is often accompanied by depression. In fact, the link is so common that there's a popular belief, even among some in the medical profession, that people who are depressed 'invent' pain. It's a view that's all the more prevalent when it comes to 'mystery' pain like fibromyalgia. The reality is that, of course, chronic pain is deeply depressing. According to the Harvard Medical School, people suffering from chronic pain are three times more likely to develop psychological problems than other people. Quite apart from the pain itself, there may be a loss of mobility, an inability to participate in normal activities, a feeling of hopelessness, a loss of self-worth, and the ever-present fear that the pain might be the result of a life-threatening condition.

Nevertheless, it *is* also true that those suffering first with depression may go on to complain of chronic pain more frequently than other people. But it's certainly not an invention. It's real and, again, according to the Harvard Medical School, the risk is about three times that of the general population.

So chronic pain can cause depression and depression can cause chronic pain. Part of the explanation is that pain and depression share common pathways in the brain. That's probably why antidepressants are also effective against pain (as we saw in Chapter 2). But there is another way of cutting into this vicious cycle and bringing it to a halt. Once again, it's exercise.

In the UK, the National Institute for Health and Clinical Excellence (NICE) recommends exercise and psychotherapy rather than antidepressants as the first line of treatment for mild depression. But it's beneficial for all types of depression. In carefully controlled trials, exercise has performed just as well as antidepressants in combating depression, but without the side effects of drugs.

Exercise is also about improving the function of just about every part of your organism. It's about feeling vital, animated, alive. It's about feeling and being healthy. And when you feel healthy you tend to feel happy rather than depressed. In fact, in many studies, good health is rated second only to marriage as a fundamental cause of happiness, particularly for older people, who don't take it for granted the way younger people do. And it works both ways. Health equals happiness and happiness equals health.

Remember this

People who exercise a little every week enjoy two extra years of life compared with the couch potatoes. And people who exercise a little more – but still only moderately – enjoy almost four extra years. Those who exercise regularly and vigorously gain as much as ten years, according to some researchers.

How exercise can protect against cancer drugs

Anthracyclines are drugs used to treat certain cancers, especially breast cancer. They're highly effective. But they come at a terrible price, causing severe heart damage by various mechanisms, including the action of free radicals on the heart muscle, the prevention of protein synthesis, calcium overload in the cells of the heart, and disturbances to cell metabolism. Beating cancer at the cost of heart disease is a cruel price to pay. But now various studies have shown that vigorous exercise inhibits all these effects.

Remember this

Here, then, are all the benefits associated with regular exercise. You will:

* increase the chemicals that combat pain
* reduce pain through improved blood supply
* feel happier
* sleep better
* have more energy
* look better
* enjoy greater self-esteem
* think more clearly (especially if you're older)
* handle stress more easily
* have a reduced risk of heart attack and stroke
* increase your levels of HDL or 'good' cholesterol
* lower your blood pressure
* increase your bone density
* boost your immune system
* enhance your sexual responsiveness
* increase your life expectancy
* protect your heart from the damaging effects of certain cancer drugs.

How much exercise?

Remember that we're primarily looking at exercise as a way of reducing pain, not improving physical fitness. So how much exercise does it take to boost those all-important chemicals? The good news is, surprisingly little. Let's take a look:

- Endorphins: the level of beta-endorphins, the chemicals the body releases to combat pain, increases five times after 12 minutes of vigorous exercise.

- Phenylethylamine (PEA): the researchers at Nottingham Trent University found that running at 70 per cent of maximum heart rate (MHR – see below) for 30 minutes increased the level of phenylacetic acid in the urine (an indicator for phenylethylamine) by 77 per cent.

- Noradrenaline/norepinephrine (NE): this increases up to ten times following eight minutes of vigorous exercise.

Remember this

It would seem that around ten minutes of vigorous exercise is already highly beneficial in terms of endorphins and NE but that PEA levels are slower to augment.

Planning your exercise regime

HOW VIGOROUS IS VIGOROUS?

Even if you're not pacing as described above, the word 'vigorous' may sound daunting, especially if you don't take any exercise at all at the moment. But, in reality, it doesn't take very long to achieve, even starting at zero.

You've probably got a pretty good idea already of what 'vigorous' feels like but let's pin it down a little more scientifically.

Step 1: calculate your maximum heart rate

Your maximum heart rate (MHR) is the level at which your heart just can't beat any faster. It can be worked out in a fitness laboratory but there is an easier and less exhausting (although less precise) way. To calculate your MHR use the following formula: 220 minus your age. For example, if you're 40 years old your MHR will be: 220 – 40 = 180.

Step 2: calculate your training heart rate

Experts argue about the percentage of MHR that provides the best training heart rate (THR). But most people are agreed that as a minimum, THR should be at least 60 per cent of MHR. Beyond 70 per cent of MHR, exercise would be classed as 'vigorous'. At 70 to 80 per cent you'd be in the zone where aerobic conditioning improves the most. You wouldn't want to go beyond 80 per cent unless you were seriously training to win races. So let's stick with the assumption that you're 40 years old and intending to exercise at the 70 per cent level. The calculation would look like this:

$(220 - 40) \times 70\% = 180 \times 70\% = 126$.

At that level you should be able to carry on a conversation – with a little bit of puffing.

Step 3: discover your resting heart rate

Your resting heart rate (RHR) is the level when you wake up in the morning and before you get out of bed. It's the measure of how well your exercise programme is going. The average RHR for men is 60 to 80 beats per minute while for women it's somewhat higher at 70 to 90 beats a minute.

If you're at 100 beats or more you're clearly not getting sufficient exercise. You should be aiming to get under 60. Athletes tend to be in the range 40 to 50. RHRs under 30 have been known.

It's not possible to say that your RHR is directly linked to pain reduction or happiness but there is an indirect link. If your RHR starts going down it's a good indication that those anti-pain and anti-depression chemicals are being produced during exercise.

Remember this

Don´t feel despondent if you have a fairly high RHR right now. In a way you´re lucky because you should be able to reduce your RHR much faster than someone who is fitter. In fact, you should see it go down by one beat per minute per week during the first ten weeks of a decent exercise programme. In other words, you'll be able to see quick results and that's very good for motivation.

Try it now

The easiest place to take your pulse is to one side of your Adam's apple. Just press gently with three fingers in the little hollow and you'll feel it. Another place is on your wrist. Turn your hand palm upwards and place the forefinger and middle finger of your other hand across your wrist at the base of your thumb. You should feel the pulse under your forefinger. Count for 15 seconds and multiply by four. However, it's not very easy taking your pulse accurately while you're exercising. A better idea is to buy a heart rate monitor with a watch-style display on your wrist. They're available quite cheaply in sports equipment shops.

HOW LONG AND HOW OFTEN?

Asking how much exercise you need is a little bit like asking how much sunshine you need or how much music you need. Come on, you've already forgotten that this is all about reducing pain and making you feel better, both physically and mentally. However, since you ask, the minimum is 20 minutes of brisk exercise three times a week (and you'll need to allow 5 minutes at either end for warming up and cooling down).

Five times a week would be better. Longer sessions, within reason, would be better still. Dr James Blumenthal carried out a study on 150 depressed people, aged 50 or over, at Duke University, North Carolina, in 1999. Not only did exercise substantially improve mood but Dr Blumenthal concluded that for each 50-minute increment of exercise, there was an accompanying 50 per cent reduction in relapse rate. So even a little is good for pain-related depression but more is better (within reason).

If you can't keep going for 20 minutes, pace yourself and do whatever you can, with the aim of building up the time.

THE RUNNER'S HIGH

The so-called 'runner's high' is somewhat extreme but if your pain allows it, it's worth aiming for. It comes on with any steady, repetitive exercise that's continued for a significant time. So you'd be far more likely to experience it in things like running, swimming, cycling and rowing than in stop-start sports such as tennis or basketball. The key is to exercise long enough to generate the necessary cocktail of chemicals, but without things getting too gruelling.

Case study

For a bet at the age of 50 I agreed to run a marathon. I had just over nine months to prepare. A marathon is 26.2 miles (42.2 km) and at that point, I swear, I couldn't run more than 26 seconds without getting out of breath. I was starting from zero. Now it's a principle of amateur preparation that you never run a marathon in training. It's just too debilitating. So when you line up for your first ever marathon you don't know for sure that you can do it. In my case, the furthest I'd run was 20 miles. The extra six miles were unknown territory. Well, I did do it and for those last few miles I was flying. I'd followed a well-established training routine and it worked perfectly. I'm not exaggerating when I say I could have carried on running without any problem. Without doubt I was experiencing the runner's high and it lasted the rest of the day. What does it feel like? Different people describe it differently. But it definitely includes a significant immunity from pain, both physical and mental, coupled with a sense of detachment and a quiet sort of happiness.

Key idea

Once you've had the runner's high you'll find it comes more and more easily. You probably won't have the time or inclination to exercise for up to an hour regularly but you could aim to have, say, a one-hour session every weekend, coupled with two to four shorter sessions during the week. During that hour-long session you should get your runner's (or swimmer's or cyclist's or whatever's) high.

WHAT TYPE OF EXERCISE?
Nowadays, there are so many fantastic ways of having fun and getting exercise without even noticing. Almost every day, it seems, someone is inventing a new sport or activity.

In terms of pain relief we're looking for two things. The first, for all kinds of pain, is getting your heart rate up sufficiently to produce those all-important endorphins. The other, for those suffering MSK pain, is improving flexibility.

Below are some suggestions but there are plenty of other things you can do – as long as, for general pain relief, you keep your heart beating at your THR for 20 minutes. The best exercise is something you enjoy and will be happy to do several times a week. It's no good relying on, say, a ski trip once a year or a game of tennis once a month. So when you're choosing, bear in mind practical considerations such as cost, distance from your home and the availability of friends.

Key idea

All the activities described below can be pursued alone. However, in terms of pain relief, you'll almost certainly be better in a group from which you can derive the additional benefits of distraction and human companionship.

Remember this

If you´re very resistant to the whole idea of exercise it´s all the more important to find an activity that really inspires you. Something that has a point to it might do the trick. For example, rather than swim up and down in a pool, you might over the course of the summer swim along a whole stretch of coastline, getting to know all the various bays. A different kind of point can come from raising money for charity through sponsored activities.

CHAIR-BASED EXERCISE

A number of studies have been carried out into chair-based exercise and they've all been extremely positive. Contrary to what might be expected, chair-based exercise actually permits a wider range of movements for some people, due to the support, stability and leverage provided by the chair. The aim though, of course, is to move to standing exercises when possible. Chair-based exercise is particularly suitable if you have:

▶ balance problems

▶ spinal problems

▶ heart problems

▶ arthritis

▶ mobility problems generally.

Initially it's best to learn the routines as part of a group. Almost certainly you should be able to find a class near you. If not, it may be possible to get a physiotherapist to visit you at home and teach you the moves. You'll need a sturdy chair without armrests on which you can sit with your thighs parallel to the floor and your feet flat on the ground. Some background music will probably help.

WALKING

Walking is a great place to start if you're not used to taking much exercise. Walk as briskly as you can manage for as long as you can manage. If you can build up to a regular 30 minutes a day, you'll be doing yourself a lot of good. With a little ingenuity you can probably incorporate your walking seamlessly into your daily life. Maybe you could walk to the station rather than driving. Maybe you could park your car further away from your place of work. And at weekends why not take a long walk in the countryside or along a beach? If you can progress from walking to jogging that would be better still.

JOGGING

Jogging is a lot of fun. The steady, rhythmical movement seems to generate more 'anti-pain' chemicals per minute than most other activities. Just think about it for a moment. Here's an exercise that:

► doesn't require any special equipment

► doesn't have to cost anything

► doesn't require any special training

► provides plenty of fresh air and sunshine out-of-doors

► can be done indoors on a machine when the weather is bad

► can be done alone or with friends

► can be done anywhere

► enhances creative thinking and permits 'meditation'

► makes progress very easy to measure.

For all those reasons, jogging is one of the very best things you can do to combat pain, as long as your joints are up to it. If not, consider swimming or cycling instead (see below).

Key idea

One of the problems is running slowly enough. Yes, slowly. Beginners tend to associate the word running with 'going fast'. Wrong. Don't rush. You're aiming for a pace you can sustain over a long period. That means going a lot slower than your sprinting pace. In fact, to begin with you should try to run no quicker than the pace of a brisk walk. If you can hardly speak you're going too fast.

Here's a programme to help you build up from zero to generating a meaningful level of anti-pain chemicals in just ten weeks. At the end of it either continue at the week ten level on three to five days or, if you really get inspired, you might like to run further.

▶ Your ten week jogging programme

Exercise for 20 minutes in accordance with the following programme plus 5 minutes warming up and 5 minutes cooling down, making a total of 30 minutes in all. Exercise at least three times a week and build up to five times. Don't run too fast – at all times you should be able to carry on a conversation.

Week	
1	Alternate 1 minute of running with 2 minutes of walking.
2	Alternate 2 minutes of running with 2 minutes of walking.
3	Alternate 3 minutes of running with 2 minutes of walking.
4	Alternate 5 minutes of running with 2 minutes of walking.
5	Alternate 6 minutes of running with 1.5 minutes of walking.
6	Alternate 8 minutes of running with 1.5 minutes of walking.
7	Run 10 minutes, walking 1.5 minutes, run 10 minutes.
8	Run 12 minutes, walk 1 minute, run 8 minutes.
9	Run 15 minutes, walk 1 minute, run 5 minutes.
10	Run 20 minutes.

Try it now

If you've got a pair of trainers and some suitable clothing why not give jogging a try right now? Walk for two minutes, run slowly for one minute, walk for two minutes, run slowly for one minute ... and so on, until 20 minutes have elapsed. Do that every other day for a week and you'll be ready to move to the next level.

SWIMMING

Swimming is the number one exercise for those with MSK pain, because the support provided by the water eases the strain on joints. If you're fit enough to keep up a steady pace then a water temperature of 26°–28° C is fine, but if you're going to take things in a more leisurely style you really need to find a pool at around 32° C, otherwise the cold water may make your pain feel worse. If your MSK pain is severe you may need to find a good-sized hydrotherapy pool where the temperature should be around 35° C.

If you're a non-swimmer at the moment, don't rule swimming out. A few lessons are all it takes to get started. If you have a problem with putting your face in the water practise doing that in a warm bath at home. You'll soon get used to it.

▶ The breast stroke is the easiest initially. The key to it from a therapeutic point of view is to make wide arm movements. These will strengthen muscles and reduce lower back pain. A narrow arm movement is more likely to strain your back.

▶ The front crawl is more demanding initially, especially in terms of breathing. Aim to keep your body flat on the water and kick just enough so that your legs remain close to the surface. Keep movements smooth. If you have a problem turning your head to breathe use a snorkel.

For either stroke be sure to wear goggles to protect your eyes from the pool chemicals and from the salt in the sea. In the breast stroke, goggles enable you to keep your head comfortably in the water between breaths, thus relieving the strain on your neck and back. Here are a few more tips:

▶ Mix up the strokes to avoid tedium in the pool if you can – crawl, breast stroke, butterfly, back stroke.

- In summer, if you live somewhere suitable, swim in a lake or the sea. To make things even more interesting, swim a different section every time so that by the end of summer you've explored a substantial area.

- Monitor your progress by keeping a record of the distance you can swim and the time; set yourself realistic goals and reward yourself when you achieve them.

- If you don't like getting water in your ears and eyes try water aerobics.

CYCLING AND SPINNING

Cycling and spinning ('cycling' indoors on a fixed bike) are great ways to get your heart into the THR zone and generate those pain-killing endorphins. And like swimming, cycling and spinning are much kinder on joints than jogging.

A bicycle, however, does impose strains of its own and needs to be correctly set up for you to avoid injury. The first step is to choose the right bike for your kind of riding. If you're staying on well-surfaced roads then a light, racing-style bicycle may suit you. However, for poor quality roads or for tracks go for a mountain bike with shock absorbers on the front forks at least. Those, combined with wider tyres, a soft saddle, handlebar covers and gloves will protect you from jarring, while the straight handlebars will prove more comfortable than the 'drops' on racing bikes. If you live in an area of very heavy traffic consider getting a bike rack for your car and transporting it to the countryside. The other way to avoid dicing with traffic (and the weather) is to get your own indoor exercise bike – or use one at a gym.

Whatever kind of bike you get, have it set up by a professional. Here are a few guidelines:

- Your back should be arched upwards like a bridge so that it flexes in response to bumps. Sitting upright is only suitable for stationary bikes. If you suffer from lumbar spinal stenosis, the leaning forward position of a normal bicycle should suit you, but if you have lumbar degenerative disc disease you may prefer a reclining bike.

- Elbows should be slightly bent to act as shock absorbers.

- Your hands should be pretty much in line with your forearms, not bent upwards (which could cause numbness).

- Your knees should go straight up and down when pedalling with no sideways movement. If you get pain in the front of your knees the saddle is probably too low, while if it's behind your knees the saddle is probably too high.

- Some experts recommend raising the saddle little by little, day by day, until it feels wrong, and then just lowering it slightly. For a mountain bike, if you can put the balls of both feet on the ground while sitting in the saddle then the saddle is definitely too low.

- Shoulders should be rolled forward.

In general, aim for a flexible 'muscle-supported posture' rather than a rigid 'skeleton-supported posture'. Initially it will be more tiring but it will be better in the long run. To allow your muscles to develop, start with rides of just two or three miles and build up gradually. Don't cause unnecessary strain by using too high a gear. Top cyclists pedal at over 100 rpm on the flat and even attain 90 rpm climbing hills. As a beginner you should aim for something like 60 – 70 rpm or roughly one complete revolution of the pedals every second. If you can't get close to that, shift to an easier gear. You'll enjoy yourself more and produce more endorphins, too.

GYM

If you join a gym, you'll have access to all kinds of exercise equipment. There's almost certain to be treadmills, rowing machines, weight-training machines, free weights and static bicycles for spinning. There may also be a swimming pool and and very likely classes in aerobic dance, yoga or similar activities.

Membership of a gym:

- doesn't require you to have any special equipment

- can be used whatever the weather

- can be visited alone or with friends

- can exercise a wide range of muscles as well as the heart/lung system

- gives access to a professional on hand to advise and motivate you

- makes progress very easy to measure.

But:

- you will require training before you can use the equipment safely

- if the gym is a long way from home you may not always feel like going

- gyms are expensive.

Try it now

Why not go *today* to a gym near you and ask to be shown around? Take a friend along.

DANCING

Dancing is the exercise for people who hate exercise. But can something that's so much fun actually reduce pain and be good for you? It certainly can. Dancing has all the benefits of jogging, burning up to 400 calories an hour, plus a few more of its own.

One of those is that you can choose a style of dancing to suit your pain. For example:

- Latin dancing is great for strengthening core muscles and reducing back pain.

- Masala Bhangra particularly works the shoulders, upper arms and upper back.

- Jazz is a good exercise for the thighs.

- Tap focuses on the calves and ankles, and will combat osteoporosis.

- Pole dancing improves flexibility (and it doesn't have to be erotic).

- 5 Rhythms, developed by Gabrielle Roth in the 1960s, incorporates Eastern philosophy and meditation with movement.

- Zumba, devised by Alberto 'Beto' Perez, is a whole collection of fitness routines to Latin-American music.

As a bonus, dancing seems to be particularly effective against dementia. In a study published in the New England Journal of Medicine, Dr Joe Verghese and colleagues studied 469 men and women who were at least 75 years old and none of whom had dementia. Five years later 124 had dementia, but those who danced frequently had a lower incidence than the others. Dancing was the only one of 11 activities analysed that had such a positive effect. Dr Verghese considers it was due to a combination of increased blood flow to the brain, less depression due to social interaction, and the challenge of memorizing steps and working with a partner.

Try it now

Put on your favourite dance music and get bopping.

DON'T FORGET FLEXIBILITY

If you're stiff and have painful joints you may not feel much like moving. And you probably think that moving would be bad for you anyway. But, in fact, lack of movement leaves your joints more painful and stiffer than they need to be. What's more, exercise strengthens the muscles and tissues around your joints, giving them more support, and reducing the likelihood of further injury. Yoga is a great way of getting those benefits and it also works directly on pain.

A team led by Dr James Carson at Oregon Health and Science University compared 28 women receiving standard fibromyalgia care with 25 women who received the same care plus yoga lessons The yoga group experienced significantly greater improvements in their condition than the non-yoga group.

In another study, 90 back pain sufferers aged 23 to 66 were split into two groups. For six months half followed standard treatment while the other half had two 90-minute sessions per week of Iyengar yoga, a style of yoga that stresses correct alignment and precise movement. At both three months and six months the yoga group was doing better than the non-yoga group.

Researchers at Duke University Medical Centre reviewed yoga studies spanning 20 years and concluded it was an effective treatment for chronic pain, especially fibromyalgia, osteoarthritis and carpal tunnel syndrome.

Keeping motivated

Knowing that exercise can reduce pain, make you happier and improve your health should be enough to make you throw down this book right now and head straight for the gym. But, unfortunately, life isn't like that. We seldom do the things that are good for us and even if we start out with the best of intentions it's all too easy to backslide. So here are a few tips on keeping motivated:

▶ Try to take your exercise regularly at a certain time every day and on your days 'off' just go for a leisurely stroll; then, when the time comes round, your body will soon start demanding that you do something active with it.

▶ If your favourite exercise is out of doors try to have an indoor back-up you can turn to in bad weather.

▶ Exercise together with friends and jolly each another along.

▶ Don't strain; take it easy and build up gradually.

▶ Keep an exercise diary and enter your distances, times, heart rates, scores or whatever; look at it from time to time and take pride in your progress.

▶ Give yourself rewards whenever you achieve a particular goal; if it's a cup you covet, then award yourself a cup – or it could be new clothes, a meal out, a massage or whatever you fancy (and can afford).

▶ Hang up a picture of yourself before you were in pain, or a poster of your ideal body: that's how you're going to look.

▶ Keep thinking of the health benefits – less pain as well as lower resting heart rate, blood pressure and weight, fewer health problems, and a potential two to ten extra years of life.

Focus points

✳ Exercise combats pain by causing the release of endorphins as well as various mood-enhancing chemicals such as phenylethylamine and norepinephrine/noradrenaline; it also increases blood flow, thus accelerating the repair of damaged tissue.

✳ Exercise is recommended by the UK's National Institute for Health and Clinical Excellence (NICE) for the treatment of mild depression, which you may suffer from if you're experiencing chronic pain.

✳ The minimum amount of exercise for 'anti-pain fitness' is 20 minutes three times a week at around 70 per cent of your maximum heart rate (MHR).

✳ Correct posture is vital in avoiding MSK pain – the Alexander technique can teach it to you.

✳ Keep motivated by writing an exercise diary and reward yourself for reaching targets.

Next step

In the next chapter we'll be looking at a radically different way of producing those pain-killing endorphins. It's laughter – and it really is no laughing matter. Science has shown that having a good laugh is seriously good for you.

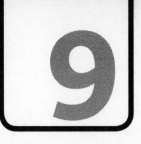

Laughter therapy

In this chapter you will learn:

- ▶ *that laughter is a serious therapy*
- ▶ *why you may get a prescription for a funny film*
- ▶ *how to laugh even when you don't feel like it.*

Life is full of misery, loneliness and suffering – and it's all over much too soon.

> Woody Allen (b. 1935), director
> and comedian.

Laughter is the tonic, the relief, the surcease for pain.

> Charlie Chaplin (1889–1977),
> comic actor and film maker.

There's an old-fashioned belief that goes like this. 'If the medicine isn't hurting, the medicine isn't working.' Well, fortunately, nothing could be further from the truth. And to underline the point, this chapter describes a pain therapy that actually works best when it makes you feel happiest. It's laughter therapy.

Many people resent the suggestion that their pain can be 'laughed away'. You may be one of them. But I'm not trivializing your pain. I take laughter therapy very seriously as an effective painkiller. Many sufferers have benefited. And I've got plenty of doctors to back me up. Here's a list of just some of the disorders the scientists say may be helped by banishing negative emotions and laughing instead: allergies, asthma, cancer, colds, depression, diabetes, flu, headaches, heart disease, hiatus hernia, hypertension, indigestion, irritable bowel syndrome, muscle pain and cramps, sexual problems, strokes and ulcers.

Although you can attend laughter therapy groups in some areas, it's also something you can do at home without spending very much or, indeed, anything at all. Laughter therapy certainly has no undesirable side effects (except for vulnerable people with certain conditions – see the warning at the end of the chapter). So why not just give it a go? You have nothing to lose and even if it has little impact on your pain, it will certainly have an impact on your quality of life. Before we start let's see what sort of a role laughter plays in your life at the moment.

Diagnostic test

For each of numbers 1 to 10 select the answer that most closely reflects your situation.

1 It's:

    a Very easy to make me laugh
    b Quite difficult to make me laugh
    c Almost impossible to make me laugh.

2 During a typical day I probably laugh:

    a At least 30 times
    b About once an hour
    c A few times
    d Barely at all.

3 I watch or listen to something funny on TV, DVD or radio or read a humorous book:

    a Every day
    b A couple of times a week
    c Rarely.

4 I tell jokes to family, friends or colleagues:

    a Most days
    b Now and then
    c Hardly ever.

5 My view of the world is:

    a It's wonderful
    b It's mostly sad with a few bright spots
    c It's in a terrible and depressing mess.

6 I believe:

    a I'm okay and other people are okay, too
    b I'm okay but it pays to be wary of other people
    c I'm not okay and feel envious of other people
    d No one is okay – and I include myself.

7 When there's a conflict with someone else I:

    a Try to diffuse it with humour
    b Give in
    c Fight to get what I want.

8 I:

    a Never bear grudges
    b Always remember an insult
    c Always try to get even.

9 I:

    a Like to lark around and be silly sometimes
    b Think it's important to treat everything seriously
    c Maintain my dignity at all times.

10 I:

    a Will certainly give laughter therapy a go
    b Would feel ridiculous laughing for no good reason
    c Will not be wasting my time on laughter therapy.

▶ **Your score**

If you scored mostly 'a': You obviously have a lot of fun and are already enjoying at least some of the benefits of laughter therapy even if you don't realize it. Keep it up and read on to discover how to use laughter in a more focused way.

If you scored mostly 'b': You tend to treat everything very seriously. That's not a terrible fault at all. In fact, if you can treat laughter therapy with the same seriousness you'll be a good subject.

If you scored mostly 'c' and 'd': You're someone who tends to feel hard done by and resentful; there's nothing jolly about your life and you're probably very resistant to the idea of laughter therapy. But, in a way, that's good because you're probably a person who could benefit enormously from it. For you it could be a big and very positive change.

Laughter really is the best medicine

Dr Lee Berk of Loma University Medical Center, California, is a man who always looks forward to going to work. For him, work is just one big laugh. He's a researcher in the relatively new discipline of psychoneuroimmunology (PNI). Not that PNI itself is anything to laugh at. But Dr Berk works in a very special niche. His job is to study the impact of humour on the human body.

PNI works on the basis that the immune system is directly linked to the brain and is affected by emotions. Generally speaking, negative emotions depress the immune system while positive emotions give it a boost.

In one experiment, Dr Berk had five men watch an hour-long comedy. Afterwards he analysed their blood and discovered something very interesting. The level of the stress hormone cortisol had fallen more rapidly than in a control group who didn't see the film. Dr Berk has also discovered that the level of the body's 'natural killer' cells (NK cells) actually increases after a humorous film. In other words, the more you laugh, the stronger your immune system. And it's not just a short-lived phenomenon. The beneficial effects of watching a humorous film for one hour lasted up to 24 hours in some individuals.

In an interview for the SuperConsciousness website, Dr Berk explained it like this: 'If I perceive an experience as stressful, my body will produce certain types of stress hormone chemicals. But, if I am laughing, my body will not create these stress hormones and we can measure those changes in the blood stream.'

In other words, the same experience can have either a detrimental, neutral or beneficial effect on the body's chemistry, depending on the way we think about it, anticipate it and perceive it. This is very much in line with cognitive therapy, which we examined in Chapter 4.

Another of Dr Berk's discoveries is that just the anticipation of 'mirthful laughter' increases beta-endorphins (the family of chemicals that elevates mood) by 27 per cent, and human growth hormone (HGH – which helps optimize immunity) by 87 per cent.

As Dr Berk told the Guardian newspaper: 'We believe the results suggest that the anticipation of a laughter eustress [positive stress] event initiates changes in neuroendocrine response prior to the event itself. From our prior studies, this modulation appears to be concomitant with mood state changes, and taken together, these would appear to carry important positive implications for wellness, disease-prevention and most certainly stress-reduction.'

So will your doctor be telling jokes? Probably not. But if he or she follows the lead of Dr Berk and his collaborator Barry Bittman MD you may well be referred not to a consultant but a comedian. Working at the Cancer Resource Center the two men have developed a tool they called SMILE (Subjective Multidimensional Interactive Laughter Evaluation). Basically, it's a computer questionnaire designed to find out exactly what kinds of things each individual finds funny. Based on that, doctors can then write a 'prescription' recommending the books and films the patient should get from the Center's library.

Remember this

In hospitals, clinics and social centres in more than 50 countries there are now over 5,000 laughter clubs. So the medical profession must be convinced that they do something good. Some were inspired by Dr Madan Kataria who created World Laughter Day in 1998. According to Dr Kataria, our great-grandparents used to laugh four times more than we do. That's hard to prove but the benefits of laughing are not. To capture those benefits Dr Kataria invented Laughter Yoga – a combination of laughter with yoga breathing – and recommends 20 minutes a day.

Case study

Probably the most influential name in 'laughter therapy' today is that of Norman Cousins, a man who was diagnosed with an extremely painful type of arthritis known as Ankylosing Spondylitis and told he had only a one in 500 chance of recovery. Till that moment he'd been content to let the doctors get on with it. That all changed when he heard the prognosis, as he recalled in his famous book *Anatomy of an Illness*. 'I felt a compulsion to get into the act,' he wrote. 'It seemed clear to me that if I was to be that one in 500 I had better be something more than a passive observer.'

His active role was to prescribe himself large doses of vitamin C and regular injections of Marx Brothers films. 'I made the joyous discovery,' he wrote, 'that ten minutes of genuine belly laughter had an anaesthetic effect and would give me at least two hours of pain-free sleep.'

Norman Cousins may sound like a crackpot but he certainly wasn't. When he died in 1990 he had a distinguished career behind him as a long-time editor of the New York-based Saturday Review, had been a leading activist for nuclear disarmament and world peace, and had spent his retirement as a faculty member of the University of California at the Los Angeles School of Medicine studying the relationship between attitude and health. His experience certainly raised the profile of 'laughter therapy' although it still isn't the universal treatment it should be.

Some doubt has now been cast on the accuracy of the original diagnosis. But that isn't the most important point. The truly important point is that he was in severe pain and that laughter reduced or even halted it, at least for a while.

Forty laughs a day

When we're young, laughter comes fairly easily. It starts as early as three weeks, according to some scientists, and certainly by four months. (Unfortunately, as far as is known, no baby ever learned to laugh before it learned to cry.)

Small children laugh around 40 times a day but as we get older we laugh less. One researcher has concluded that adults in the West laugh an average of just 17 times a day. That's not actually very much. Little more than once an hour, in fact. I'm aiming to get you laughing at least those 40 times a day you enjoyed as a child.

Laughter and pain

So laughing is good for you. It can improve your health and in so doing it may indirectly reduce your pain. But can it actually achieve anything directly? Yes it can. In 1987, Texas Tech psychologist Rosemary Cogan used the discomfort of a pressure cuff to test the effect of laughter in pain management. She divided volunteers into five groups. One group listened to a humorous Bill Cosby tape, another heard Edgar Allen Poe, a third group heard a lecture, a fourth worked on a maths problem and the fifth did nothing at all. The result was that those who listened to the humorous tape were able to tolerate 20 per cent more pain than any of the others. That was under experimental conditions. But James Rotton Ph.D of Florida International University found much the same in the real world. He noted that orthopaedic surgery patients who watched humorous films requested fewer painkillers and tranquillizers than those who didn't watch them.

How does it work? One clue has come from a study by Edward Smith, a psychologist at Columbia University, who compared brain images of 40 volunteers who had recently been dumped by their partners. He found that the neural pathways that respond to rejection overlapped with those that responded to physical pain. The conclusion is that the two types of pain are reinforcing. If you're in physical pain your emotional pain may be more intense and if you're in emotional pain your physical pain may be more intense. As to the specific role of laughter, research at Stanford University using fMRI (functional magnetic resonance imaging) shows that when we laugh an area of the limbic system called the nucleus accumbens is very active and produces dopamine. It's the same area that lights up during sex as well as during moderate exercise, activities that also reduce pain.

Case study

Pamela lived in a nursing home where, in 2009, 36 elderly men and women agreed to take part in an eight-week programme of laughter therapy. In the first one-hour session she and the other participants created collections of all the things they found funny – jokes, cartoons, photographs, books, audio tapes, films and their own personal recollections. Each of the following seven hour-long sessions began with joke-telling and continued with laughter exercises, funny games and the recounting of funny stories. At the end of the eight-week period, Pamela's pain score had fallen from 5.19 to 3.22 and, what's more, her loneliness score had fallen from 42.50 to 39.44, while her happiness score had gone up from 16.19 to 23.03 and her life satisfaction score from 10.50 to 12.67.

Try it now

One special way of dealing with pain through laughter is to reframe it. This would be known in NLP (see Chapter 3) as a 'meaning' or 'content' reframe. The way it works is to do something to increase the pain a little and then laugh. It sounds ridiculous but it can help. For example, if you have an arthritic joint move it until it just hurts and then give it your best chortle. Pain. Laugh. Pain. Laugh. Pain. Laugh. Keep doing it until the pain doesn't seem so bad. The laughter doesn't necessarily make the pain go away but it can change the way your brain deals with it. Milton Erickson, whose hypnotic techniques we also looked at in Chapter 3, once helped an amputee suffering phantom limb pain simply by planting the suggestion that a phantom limb could equally be a source of pleasure. Laughter can achieve the same effect of reprogramming the brain.

Key idea

There are people who enjoy pain. We call them masochists. Something has happened in their brains to confuse pleasure and pain signals. Which proves that your brain can be reprogrammed through laughter to feel pain less keenly.

WHAT HAPPENS WHEN YOU LAUGH?

Let's first of all trace what happens in the brain when you hear a good joke.

- An electrical wave moves through the cerebral cortex (the largest part of the brain) within less than half a second of seeing or hearing something potentially funny.

- The left side of the cortex analyses the joke or situation.

- Activity increases in the frontal lobe.

- The occipital lobe processes any visual signals.

- The right hemisphere of the cortex is where you 'get' the joke.

- The most 'primitive' part of the brain – the limbic system (especially amygdala and hippocampus) – is involved in the emotional response.

- The hypothalamus is involved in the production of loud, uncontrollable laughter.

So your brain is getting a good workout, for a start.

In turn, the laughter:

- reduces pain, possibly by the production of endorphins but certainly through relaxation and distraction

- lowers stress hormones, including cortisol

- relaxes the body

- speeds recovery from surgery, especially for children

- increases the disease-fighting protein Gamma-interferon

- increases T-cells and B-cells which make disease-fighting antibodies

- increases immunoglobulins (antibodies) A, M and G, which defend the body from pathogens

- increases Complement 3, which helps antibodies pierce defective or infected cells in order to destroy them

- benefits anyone suffering from diabetes because it lowers blood sugar

- benefits the heart

- lowers blood pressure (after an initial increase)

- strengthens abdominal muscles

- flushes water vapour from the lungs.

Remember this

Given all its benefits, laughter may do more than reduce your pain. Depending on what your diagnosis is, laughter might actually improve your underlying condition, or even cure it.

Try it now

What kind of humour makes you laugh out loud? Which actor or comedian is the funniest person you know of? Well, get yourself a handful of DVDs that are pretty much guaranteed to have you rolling around and watch half an hour at a time. Don't act like a critic. Just give in to it.

Fake it till you make it

So you're now persuaded of the benefits of laughter. But supposing you just don't find anything very funny. What then?

Here's the incredible thing. Our hormonal system isn't very good at telling the difference between real laughter and fake laughter. In effect, pretending that you find something funny is almost as effective as actually finding it funny. You could say it's a sort of laughter placebo. The catchphrase for laughter therapists is this: Fake it till you make it.

GET INTO TRAINING

If you're going to laugh more than ever before you've got to get into training. If you were strengthening your biceps you'd pick up weights even though you didn't actually want them, in other words, for no reason. It's the same with smiling and laughter. You've got to learn to smile for no reason. You've got to learn to laugh for no reason.

Then, in the same way that you can become capable of lifting heavier and heavier weights, so you can become capable of smiling and laughing in 'heavier and heavier' situations.

I learned this lesson years ago from a woman who taught children with a wide range of disabilities. She was always smiling, always laughing in the midst of difficulties and, at first, it annoyed me. How could everything seem so funny to her? How could she be so insensitive to all the problems of her pupils, let alone the rest of the world? It seemed to be a kind of madness.

One day, perhaps reading my mind, she explained it to me. Many of her pupils with quite severe disabilities were nevertheless happy. How could she not be happy with all the advantages she had? And then I saw very clearly my own disability. She had pupils who, for example, couldn't walk without callipers. In my case, I couldn't be happy, couldn't laugh, unless I, too, was provided with artificial assistance.

She wasn't mad at all. She was one of the few sane people. It's the rest of us who are mad. If we need assistance to laugh and be happy then we, too, are disabled. So practise your unassisted laughing and cure your disability.

Key idea

The success of laughter therapy brings us back yet again to the connection between emotion and pain. This isn't surprising because we now know that negative emotion caused by pain is processed in the same area of the brain as negative emotion caused by unpleasant or sad events. Indeed, some painkillers actually reduce emotional pain just as they do physical pain.

Try it now

I want you to laugh, right now, for no reason. No matter where you are, just do it. Don't worry about people thinking you're crazy – they'll assume you're laughing at something in the book. Better still, if there's no one else around try a whole range of laughs from a snigger through a chesty rumble to a maniacal cackle. Keep it up for several minutes because it takes a while for the body to respond.

▶ Warning – laughing can sometimes be a bad thing

There are just a few medical conditions that could be made worse by too much laughing. If you're asthmatic, laughing just might trigger an attack. It can also be bad for anyone with a serious heart condition, a hernia, severe piles, certain eye problems, and anyone who has just undergone abdominal surgery.

Focus points

* Frequent, daily laughter can help with a wide range of health problems.
* After a good bout of laughing your sensitivity to pain will go down by about a fifth.
* Even fake laughter has a beneficial effect.
* Emotional pain increases sensitivity to physical pain.
* By laughing at your pain you can reprogram your brain to be less sensitive to it.

Next step

Having a good laugh is a pretty agreeable way of reducing pain and one of the most ancient. In the next chapter we'll be taking a look at some of the most modern pain-reduction methods, Transcutaneous Electrical Nerve Stimulation (TENS) and ultrasound.

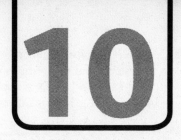

Electrical and ultrasound therapy

In this chapter you will learn:

▶ *how a cheap electrical device might turn down your pain*

▶ *how sound waves can 'massage' you deep inside*

▶ *how you can accelerate the absorption of painkilling creams.*

Pain is the most common symptom that takes patients to a physician, but no one has specialized in pain management.

Dr Norman Shealy (b. 1932), inventor of Transcutaneous Electrical Nerve Stimulation (TENS), speaking in 1970.

Technology is bringing effective drug-free pain relief ever closer. For the moment techniques such as transcranial direct current stimulation (tDCS) are mostly experimental but it's probable that in one or two decades it will be possible to switch pain off as easily as clicking a computer mouse. But we're not there yet. For the moment, there are two interesting technologies you can use at home. Both are controversial but they're worth a go. They are:

▶ Transcutaneous Electrical Nerve Stimulation (TENS). Available since the 1970s, TENS works by delivering electrical impulses via pads attached to the skin.

▶ Ultrasound. Well known as a diagnostic tool, ultrasound has been used experimentally for pain relief since the 1960s, but it's only recently that there's been any impetus behind the development of ultrasound as a standard pain relief technique.

Many users are highly satisfied with their TENS and ultrasound units and are convinced their pain has been reduced or stopped altogether by them. On the other hand, properly controlled scientific studies have found them to be no better than placebo. All that can be said is that if other therapies have failed, or not been suitable for some reason, you have nothing to lose (except a fairly small amount of money) by trying them. They may work in your case.

Will they be suitable for you? Take this test:

Diagnostic test

1 Are your painkillers causing unpleasant side effects?

2 Do you prefer not to take medicaments?

3 Are you pregnant and wanting a natural birth without chemical painkillers?

4 Are you allergic to NSAIDs?

5 Are you suffering chronic pain that resists analgesics?

6 Are you open to new technologies?

7 Are you willing to spend all or part of the day with wires stuck to your body?

8 Are you the kind of person who enjoys experimenting?

9 Are you drawn to alternative/complementary therapies?

10 Do you like the idea of being in control of your own pain relief?

▶ **Your score**

The more times you answered 'yes' the more likely you are to benefit from TENS and/or ultrasound. If you answered 'no' to pretty much everything, they may not work for you.

TENS

TENS machines are little boxes about the size of smart phones which send electrical impulses to the body via pads stuck to the skin. It's claimed they work through three mechanisms:

▶ They cause the body to produce endorphins, its own natural painkillers

▶ They interfere with or block pain messages

▶ They distract from the sensation of pain.

People use the machines in various ways. Some use them only when they have a crisis. Some use them at regular intervals throughout the day. Some use them only for particularly painful activities. And some have them on almost constantly.

You should be able to try a TENS machine at a pain clinic for a short while and in some cases you may also be able to take a machine home to try for four to six weeks. However, TENS machines can be bought so cheaply nowadays that you may think it worth having one in the house for general use.

HOW GOOD IS TENS?

Scientific studies have often been unfavourable to TENS but a review of comments on the internet found users reporting benefits in a wide range of conditions including not only MSK pain but also tension headaches, migraine and fibromyalgia. Generally the pain-killing effect doesn't last very long after the machine has been switched off but some users with MSK pain do report a permanent cure. How that can be is not clear but in all probability the immediate pain relief restores mobility which in turn improves blood flow.

CHOOSING A TENS MACHINE

Cheaper machines tend to have fixed settings. If you can afford it, buy a machine that allows you to choose the number of pulses per second (frequency), the length of each pulse, and the mode (constant, modulation or burst modes). Two electrodes are enough but four are better. TENS machines also exist in the form of wands and pens which many find useful for pains in fingers, toes and other very specific places – but they do require users to hold them all the time.

Case study

'I take daily medication for chronic pain but sometimes it breaks through and that's when I use my TENS machine. I've found it particularly useful for back and neck pain and migraines but I've also tried it for period pain and irritable bowel syndrome and it helps with those conditions, too. It took me a while to find the right pad positions for me. You've got to be persistent.' Kelly (28)

Key idea

It is safe to keep the machine on for lengthy periods. Some users keep theirs on all the time they are awake but do place the electrodes in a different position every morning to prevent the skin becoming sore.

HOW TO USE A TENS MACHINE

Getting the best out of a TENS machine requires quite a bit of experimentation in terms of settings and the placement of the electrodes. If you don't experience any pain relief initially, persist with different electrode placements and different settings. Don't assume that TENS is ineffective in your case until you've tried all the possibilities.

Machines vary in the options they offer but here are some general rules:

1 Test the battery to make sure it is sufficiently charged. If there is no battery check facility, hold the electrodes between your fingers and switch on – you should feel a tingling sensation.

2 Clean the skin where you intend to place the electrodes with alcohol (surgical spirit) and then dry it.

3 If you have rubber non-adhesive electrodes put a thin layer of gel on the bottom of each one – this makes them stick and improves the electrical contact. If you have self-adhesive electrodes don't use gel.

4 Place the electrodes on your skin – if the wires detach from the electrodes it will be easier if you detach them. The pads should be either side of the pain and at least one inch (2.5 cm) apart. Note that if you have a four electrode machine the electrodes should be placed in pairs – the current will flow from one of the pair to the other.

5 Using sticky tape over the electrode will ensure a good contact and is essential if you're going to be moving around.

6 Connect the wires to the electrodes (if disconnected).

7 For acute pain and for your first try, choose constant stimulation, a pulse rate (frequency) of 80 – 100 Hz, and a pulse duration of 100 – 200 microseconds.

8 For muscle relaxation and if setting 1 is insufficient, choose modulation (the frequency varies), a pulse rate (frequency) of 60 – 100 Hz and a pulse duration of 100 – 200 microseconds.

9 For chronic pain and if settings 1 and 2 were insufficient, choose burst mode, a pulse rate (frequency) of 2 – 10 Hz and a pulse duration of 100 – 200 microseconds.

10 After a few minutes the sensation may appear to lessen (known as 'accommodation') and you should then adjust the settings again.

When the session is over, wash the skin. If you use rubber pads clean the gel off with soap and water. Do not wash self-adhesive pads.

The sensations you feel are an indication of the nerves you're working on:

▶ Pins and needles that are not painful – you're stimulating the large, non-pain nerves.

▶ Pins and needles that are painful – you're stimulating the small skin sensation nerves.

▶ Muscles twitching - you're stimulating the small nerves coming from the muscles.

Do not place electrodes:

▶ On broken skin

▶ On areas that are numb

▶ On areas that are hypersensitive

▶ On the front of the neck

▶ On the eyes

▶ One on the chest and one on the back.

Key idea

If it's not physically possible to stick the electrodes close to the area of pain it may still be effective to use them further along the same nerve. Get a diagram of the nerves in the body to work out the best alternative position.

Remember this

Note that, over the long term, the body can become habituated to TENS and the treatment may become less effective. In that case you may restore relief by using different settings and electrode placements. If not, take a break from the machine. Hopefully its effectiveness will return.

SIDE EFFECTS

There are few side effects with TENS. Some people have an allergic reaction to the pads. You must not use a TENS machine if you wear a pacemaker or are pregnant (except for the delivery – see 'TENS in labour' below). If you have heart problems speak to your doctor first. Do not place electrodes on your head or neck if you have epilepsy or suffer from convulsions.

TENS IN LABOUR

TENS has become a popular method of pain relief for giving birth. As with other uses, the scientific studies are not very positive but many individual women, including some who have given birth both with and without TENS, are certain of the benefits. Any four-pad TENS machine is suitable for labour but you may prefer one of the purpose-designed models that has a 'booster' button for when contractions are at their most painful.

Once labour is under way you won't feel much like experimenting with your TENS machine so become completely familiar with it beforehand. If you have a birth partner, he or she should learn all about the machine and take care of setting it up. The usual way of using TENS for labour is to place one pair of pads either side of your spine just below the level of your bra strap. The second pair should be placed either side of your spine just above the buttocks. Practise this beforehand but don't switch the machine on as it shouldn't be used until labour begins.

Once labour begins, however, the pads should be put in position and the machine switched on. As always you may need to experiment a little with the placement of the pads. Once you find the best spots it may be a good idea to use sticky tape to secure them firmly.

....
Remember this

You shouldn't use TENS if you're less than 37 weeks pregnant. And you can't use it in a birthing pool (or in the bath or shower).
....

Ultrasound

Ultrasound is more difficult to use effectively at home than TENS and user experience is quite variable. Many are disconcerted that their ultrasound device doesn't appear to do anything. If you buy a home unit you'll discover that it makes no noise and produces no discernible vibrations. The explanation is that ultrasound is outside the range of human hearing. This tends to make users wary of being duped and possibly impacts on the feedback they give.

As regards the scientific evidence, Valma J. Robertson and Kerry G. Baker examined 35 randomized controlled trials (RCTs) between 1975 and 1999 and found only 10 to be of an acceptable standard. Of those, two concluded that ultrasound was better than placebo for certain problems while eight concluded that it wasn't.

One positive study, led by Meltem Esenyel MD at Vakif Gureba Teaching Hospital in Istanbul, concluded that ultrasound was as effective as trigger point injections for the treatment of myofascial pain (pain in the connective tissue that covers muscles). The study, however, did not control for the placebo effect.

A study led by Anil Khanna and published in the British Medical Bulletin in 2008 concluded that a type of ultrasound known as low-intensity pulsed ultrasound (LIPUS) promoted healing in soft tissues such as inter-vertebral discs and cartilage.

Key idea

The use of ultrasound is widespread in sports physiotherapy.

WHAT KINDS OF PAIN CAN BE TREATED WITH ULTRASOUND?

Manufacturers of home ultrasound equipment claim it can relieve pain caused by inflammation and reduced circulation. It's said to be particularly suitable for injuries to tendons, ligaments and muscles and for the treatment of conditions such as arthritis, bursitis, carpal tunnel syndrome and swollen discs. Used on the back of the neck it may also relieve tension headaches and migraines. It's not suitable for pain in any organs such as the stomach or kidneys.

HOW DOES ULTRASOUND WORK?

Ultrasound waves have the ability to penetrate quite deeply into tissues where they cause heat. It's claimed the heat releases tension and improves blood flow, relieving pain and speeding recovery.

HOW DO I CHOOSE AN ULTRASOUND MACHINE?

Units generally operate at 800,000 Hz to 2,000,000 Hz, well above the level that can be detected by the human ear (around 20,000 Hz). The lower the frequency the deeper the penetration. Generally, 1,000,000 Hz is considered the optimum for therapy.

Remember this

Power output is measured in watts per square centimetre. Home models tend to have less power than professional models but that's fine because better results are obtained with lower power and longer sessions rather than with high power and short sessions. A model with a power output of 1 watt per square centimetre is fine.

HOW DO I USE MY ULTRASOUND MACHINE?

You'll need a special ultrasound gel, or 'coupling agent', which is spread on the skin over the area to be treated. Without the coupling agent the sound waves will not be transmitted and the therapy will be completely ineffective. For most kinds of pain the optimum treatment is said to be 3 to 10 minutes two to four times a day. For that reason a home unit is far more practical than professional treatment. You won't feel very much during an ultrasound session and it certainly shouldn't cause any pain.

USING ULTRASOUND FOR DRUG DELIVERY

In place of the standard coupling agents it's possible to buy analgesic gels, specially formulated to transmit ultrasound. Studies show that suitable topical analgesics are absorbed more efficiently in combination with ultrasound than they are with normal massage in a process known as phonophoresis (or sonophoresis).

It seems the heating effect of the ultrasound increases the kinetic energy of the molecules in the drug and also in the cell membranes, dilates hair follicles and sweat glands which act as points of entry, and increases circulation in the area. All of this enhances the ability of the drug molecules to diffuse through the stratum corneum (the outer layer of the skin) and into the capillary network in the dermis.

It's important to be sure that your chosen analgesic gel does, indeed, transmit ultrasound effectively. A study published in 2001, (J. William Myrer, Gary J. Measom, Gilbert W. Fellingham) showed that two analgesic gels, Nature's Chemist and Biofreeze, could be mixed 1:1 with a standard ultrasound gel (Aquasonic 100), without reducing the warming efficiency of ultrasound in the soft tissues. However, other topical analgesics have performed poorly as coupling agents. For up-to-date advice put 'ultrasound analgesic gel' into your internet search engine.

The benefit of phonophoresis is that the drug is delivered where it's needed, or at least close to the problem area, whereas an oral medicine drugs the entire body. Having said that, there will always be some systemic effect because the drug will enter the bloodstream.

In one study as long ago as 1967 (Griffin, J.E., Echternach, J.L., Price, R.E.), hydrocortisone photophoresis was given once a week for three weeks for patients with osteoarthritis, periarticular arthritis, or joint and muscle problems. Sixty-eight per cent had a decrease in pain and an increase in range of motion compared with only 25 per cent who received the same ultrasound treatment with a placebo drug.

IS ULTRASOUND DANGEROUS?

Ultrasound is safe when used as intended. It shouldn't be used:

▶ On the abdomen, pelvic region or lower back in women who are pregnant or menstruating

▶ Over internal organs

▶ On the front of the neck

▶ On broken skin

▶ Over fractures which haven't healed yet

▶ Around the eyes

▶ Around the breasts or genitals

▶ Over malignant tumours or suspected tumours

▶ Over areas with impaired sensation

▶ Over plastic implants

▶ Over areas that have had cortisone injections in the past 30 days

▶ On children without medical advice

▶ On those suffering from phlebitis, deep vein thrombosis, haemophilia, spina bifida, or wearing pace-makers.

TENS and ultrasound for fibromyalgia

One exciting development could be the use of TENS together with ultrasound as a combination therapy, a strategy that has been researched by Felipe Azevendo Moretti at the Universidade Federal in Sao Paulo.

Before his study began, patients were asked to rate their level of pain on the first day of the trial as well as over the preceding week on a scale of 1 to 10 (with 10 being the worst possible). They were also asked about the number of tender points, their quality of their sleep, and their quality of life.

Over a 12 week period, half the patients received one session per week and the other half received two per week. At the end of the trial they were again asked to rate the same factors.

The results seem impressive. For those receiving once-weekly treatments, average pain score fell from 7.6 on the first day of the trial to 3.1 at the end of the trial, a reduction of better than 50 per cent. As regards the pain experienced in the week before the trial compared to the last seven days of the trial, the results were even more dramatic, tumbling from 9.5 to 3.3. Sleep quality and quality of life improved by more than a third and the number of tender points fell by half. Results for the twice-weekly sessions were similar, so on the basis of this trial it seems that having the combined treatment just once a week is sufficient for many conditions. However, it has to be said the methodology of the Sao Paulo trial does not convince everyone.

Focus points

* Transcutaneous Electrical Nerve Stimulation (TENS) is said to block pain signals and cause the body to produce pain-killing endorphins.
* Ultrasound machines send high-frequency sound waves deep into the body where, it is claimed, they heat tissue, relax tension, restore blood flow and reduce pain.
* Ultrasound can be used as a treatment on its own or as a way of delivering drugs, especially analgesics.
* TENS and ultrasound can be used in combination, a technique that, according to one trial, has proven especially useful for fibromyalgia.
* Well-conducted scientific studies mostly find TENS and ultrasound to be no better than placebo, but many users report impressive pain reduction.

Next step

This chapter brings to an end this review of the many possible treatments for acute and chronic pain of all sorts. In the next chapter you'll find advice on creating a treatment programme for your particular pain.

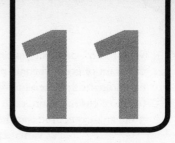

Your pain reduction programme

In this chapter you will learn:

▶ *how to tackle common painful conditions*
▶ *how to get a fast fix*
▶ *how to develop a long-term pain reduction programme.*

With today's advances in brain imaging we can see that the brain of every chronic pain patient is structurally and psychologically different. We found that there are different forms of chronic pain, each with their unique brain imprint. You can't expect to treat them all in the same way.'

Vania Apkarian, chronic pain researcher,
Northwestern University, Illinois, USA.

So you've finished reading about the various ways of tackling pain. Now it's time to take action. But don't just seize on one therapy because you like the sound of it or because it seems easy. Be methodical. So often, no one single thing will be a cure. You need to tackle your pain in every possible way simultaneously.

Your first step should be to draw up a programme. Below I give examples for some of the commonest kinds of pain and the way each of them can be tackled. If your type of pain is one of the ten I've chosen then I've done the job for you. Otherwise, make a list of the various things you'll do, and the things you'll stop doing, and implement it.

Naturally, you want a fast fix. Who doesn't? But don't leave it at that. A fast fix is often a short-term fix. In order to stop the pain permanently you need a long-term programme.

Back pain

Back pain is a huge problem, affecting at least a fifth of adult Westerners at any given moment. In a lifetime, at least two-thirds of Westerners will suffer significant back pain. In one survey in Australia, of those people who reported pain the majority reported back pain.

It may seem that chronic back pain is essentially a mechanical problem that requires surgery. But most doctors now agree that surgery should only ever be a last resort. Don't agree to surgery until you've tried everything else. The fundamental cause of most back problems is restricted blood flow in the arteries that serve the spine. That's what you have to sort out. Even children suffer and it's been estimated that by the age of 20 about 10 per cent of Westerners already have serious blockages.

Fast fix:

▶ Take non-specific anti-inflammatory drugs (Chapter 2) or, in a severe case, ask your doctor for a transforaminal epidural injection of corticosteroid (Chapter 2).

▶ A hot water bottle can help a lot.

Long-term programme:

▶ Change your attitude to the limitations of back pain (Chapters 3 and 4).

▶ Improve the circulation. Self-treatments to do that include reducing stress (Chapter 4), reducing fat in the diet (Chapter 5), heat and massage (Chapter 7), and improved posture and exercise (Chapter 8).

▶ Laughter always helps (Chapter 9).

Key idea

Wear a back support when lifting. America's National Institute of Occupational Safety and Health has concluded that back supports do not prevent injuries, a view supported by a study of 300 airline cargo loaders. But a 2009 study of 197 sufferers of subacute low back pain concluded that a brace improved the range of motion and reduced pain and therefore the need for medication. So a brace is worth trying.

Fibromyalgia

Fibromyalgia (from the Latin *fibro*, meaning fibrous tissue, and the Greek words *myo*, meaning muscle, and *algos*, meaning pain) is a somewhat mysterious condition resulting in deep muscle pain in various parts of the body, extreme sensitivity to touch, fatigue, sleep disturbance and depression. There may be other related problems, too.

Fibromyalgia is often wrongly diagnosed. It's not fibromyalgia if fewer than 11 of 18 tender points are involved. The 18 are:

▶ Two in the front of the neck

▶ Two in the back of the neck

- Four at the shoulders
- Two on the upper chest
- Two in the elbow region
- Two on the inside of the knees
- Two at the upper buttocks
- Two on the outside of the upper thighs, just below the buttocks.

If at least 11 of these 18 points hurt when pressed with a finger then the diagnosis is fibromyalgia.

Fast fix:

- Your doctor may prescribe an opioid painkiller, a nerve membrane stabilizer, and an antidepressant (Chapter 2). Flupirtine, an analgesic available in various countries but not, at the time of writing, in either the UK or the USA, has shown great promise in early trials for fibromyalgia (Chapter 2). Four women sufferers in Massachusetts, all of whom had tried multiple treatments without success, were put on flupirtine. Three of the women enjoyed a dramatic improvement in all symptoms and the fourth experienced moderate relief from joint pain and sleep disturbance.

Long-term programme:

- Mind Controlled Analgesia (Chapters 3 and 4). If you know or suspect you have been the victim of abuse psychotherapy may help. Dr John Sarno controversially sees fibromyalgia as a manifestation of tension myositis syndrome (TMS – see Chapter 4).

- Regular exercise (Chapter 8). You may not feel like it but there's plenty of evidence that exercise improves all fibromyalgia symptoms. Start today by doing something, however small. It could just be walking up the stairs or taking a stroll around the garden. Every day try to do just a little more.

- Laughter always helps (Chapter 9).

Headaches

Headaches are one of the commonest kinds of pain. They can take many forms and have many causes but most of them can be categorized as:

► Tension-type headaches

► Cluster headaches

► Migraine headaches.

► **Fast fix:**

► A huge range of painkilling drugs is available (Chapter 2)

► A huge range of prophylactics (preventive drugs) is available (Chapter 2).

► **Long-term programme:**

► The best long-term solution is to discover what things trigger your headaches and circumvent them if at all possible. Common triggers for headaches include:

  ▷ Food. Certain foods are well-known to trigger headaches in susceptible people (Chapter 5). Note that a headache or migraine may be linked to food eaten as long ago as the previous day.

  ▷ Skipping a meal or becoming dehydrated.

  ▷ Cold food and drink. Cold food and drink can cause a sharp pain in the forehead. Fortunately this type of headache usually passes within a couple of minutes.

▷ Emotional problems often lead to headaches and migraines. A study of 1,856 Brazilian children found a particularly marked correlation. It seems that internalizing problems is the real culprit. Speak to someone about your emotional problems and try the techniques in Chapters 3 and 4.

▷ Stress often leads to headaches, especially tension headaches. Try the techniques in Chapters 3 and 4, learn to relax (Chapter 6) and try to laugh at things (Chapter 9).

▷ But relaxation itself can cause problems. After, say, a stressful week at work a lie-in on Saturday or Sunday can result in a headache due to changes in hormones and neurotransmitters. It may be best to forego it.

▷ Anger causes tension in the muscles of the neck and shoulders leading to the sensation of constriction around the forehead. See Chapters 3 and 4 for techniques such as NLP, CBT and self-hypnosis that can be adapted for anger management.

▷ Poor posture. Some lessons in the Alexander Technique may solve this (Chapter 8). Avoid staying in one position for too long. Get up and move around at least once an hour.

▷ Eye strain. Have your eyes checked. If the pressure is too high your ophthalmologist may prescribe drops but daily doses of two grams of vitamin C are also effective for some people – and vitamin C has other benefits, too.

▷ Smells. Strong perfumes in scent, soap, deodorants, cleaning products and so on trigger headaches in some people. Avoid them.

▷ Grinding teeth. If you grind your teeth in your sleep you may wake up with a headache, as well as have dental problems. The best way to stop it is to train yourself to keep your jaw relaxed during the day. Avoid stress (Chapter 6). Avoid caffeine and alcohol in the evening.

▷ Glare. The glare of bright lights is a trigger for some people, especially if it comes from fluorescent tubes which flicker. Change the lighting, if you can. Sunglasses will help out of doors.

▷ Sex. Some unfortunate people get headaches during or after sex. It could be due to neck muscles or it could also be hormonal. If you're a man you may find that non-ejaculatory sex solves the problem.

▷ The weather. Some people really can predict the weather by the pain in their heads. It's all to do with changing pressure. There's no way of avoiding this one.

▶ Laughter always helps (Chapter 9).

▶ Transcutaneous electrical nerve stimulation (TENS). In one study (Seymour Solomon MD, Karen M. Guglielmo BS,) 55 per cent of patients with migraine or muscle contraction headache said pain was reduced by TENS, compared with only 18 per cent who noted an improvement on placebo (Chapter 10).

Remember this

The vast majority of headaches are not life-threatening. However, you should seek urgent medical attention if your headache:

✳ Starts suddenly and becomes agonizing within seconds or minutes

✳ Occurs with fever and/or stiff neck and is severe

✳ Occurs together with personality changes, confusion, seizure or passing out

✳ Occurs with weakness, numbness and vision problems and you haven't previously been diagnosed with migraine.

Key idea

Here's a quick tip that works for some tension headaches. While sitting upright, take a small, clean coin and place it on your forehead just above your nose. Relax and breathe from your belly. With one finger slide it up a little further until you sense that it's nestling in a tiny depression approximately in the middle of your forehead. Take your finger away. If you keep the muscles of your forehead relaxed the coin will remain in place. With your hands resting on your knees and your eyes closed, continue relaxed breathing. If you contract the muscles of your forehead the coin will fall off. It thus acts as a biofeedback device for avoiding forehead tension. If you can keep the coin in place for a while there's a good chance your tension headache will go.

Heartburn, gastroesophageal reflux disease (GERD) and ulcers

About a fifth of Westerners suffer from heartburn about once a week. It has nothing to do with the heart, although it may feel like it. It's caused by acid from the stomach splashing up into the oesophagus. There's a valve to prevent that happening but sometimes it doesn't close as tightly as it should.

If you regularly have heartburn twice a week or more, a doctor would consider you were suffering from gastroesophageal reflux disease (GERD).

The pain of peptic ulcers is caused by the action of acid on areas of the stomach or duodenum where there's a hole in the protective coating. So these three conditions have things in common.

▶ **Fast fix:**

▶ Take antacids (to combat stomach acid) or ask your doctor about proton pump inhibitors and H_2 antagonists which, through different mechanisms, reduce gastric acid production.

▶ **Long-term programme:**

You need a certain strength of stomach acid for the proper digestion of food, otherwise, undigested proteins cause an increased risk of developing allergies. That's just one of the reasons it's best to avoid long-term use of acid-reducing pills. A proper programme to restore the health of your digestive tract is what's needed.

▶ Excess acid may also be the result of an overgrowth of the bacterium *Helicobacter pylori* which can live in the stomach. A course of antibiotics (usually two types) together with a proton pump inhibitor should take care of it. Note that when the treatment is over, coming off the proton pump inhibitor may cause renewed heartburn due to the rebound effect. The solution is to taper down over a couple of weeks, rather than stop abruptly. Researchers at the John Hopkins University in Baltimore and the National Center for Scientific Research in Paris have demonstrated, in the lab at least, that cruciferous vegetables containing sulforaphane, such as broccoli, cabbage and kale, can destroy the bacterium. A diet high in these vegetables will help prevent *H. pylori* reaching critical levels again.

▶ The most important step for your gastrointestinal health, aside from tackling *H. pylori*, is to identify and avoid foods that trigger heartburn. Everyone is different in this but common triggers are fatty foods, tomato sauce, chocolate, mint, garlic, onions, caffeine and alcohol. Some of these are also triggers for other painful conditions (Chapter 5). Whatever you eat, eat less more often – don't ever feel you 'couldn't eat another thing'.

▶ Obesity is one of the risk factors for GERD so keeping to a healthy weight would be a good idea.

▶ Slippery elm may help (Chapter 5).

▶ Avoiding stress and learning to relax may help (Chapter 6).

▶ Acupuncture may help (Chapter 7).

▶ Don't lie down or go to bed within three hours of eating a meal. If you suffer from acid reflux at night raise the head of your bed by six to nine inches (15 – 23 cm) or insert a wedge (from a medical supply company) under the mattress. Using additional pillows is far less effective.

▶ Don't smoke.

▶ Don't wear tight clothing around your abdomen.

Hiatus hernia

The pain that sometimes results from a hiatus hernia can be severe. It comes right in the middle of the chest and can seem like a heart attack. The problem is due to enlargement of the opening in the diaphragm through which the oesophagus reaches the stomach. Quite often the enlargement causes no symptoms at all. However, it sometimes happens that the top of the stomach pushes up through the opening and becomes stuck. As a result, acid from the stomach can splash up into the oesophagus, causing burning. In addition, the top of the stomach is crushed, while at the same time the opening in the diaphragm is unnaturally distended. This combination can result in a pain that can bring tough men to their knees.

▶ **Fast fix:**

This is actually a mechanical problem and you can halt the pain in a simple mechanical way. You need to get your stomach back down where it should be.

▶ One way to do that is to repeatedly jump off, say, the bottom step of a staircase, landing with a good flat-footed thud. If your stomach is empty it will help to drink a couple of mugs of warm water. The warmth will relax things and the weight, as you jump, will help return the stomach to where it should be.

An alternative is to try to manipulate your stomach back into place with your hands:

▶ With the tips of the fingers of your right hand find the bottom of your ribcage in the centre of your chest.

▶ Slide your hand about the width of two fingers towards your left side, along the bottom of your lowest rib. (The stomach goes right across your abdomen but your liver can get in the way on your right side.)

▶ As you breathe out, push your fingertips horizontally inwards under the ribs and then downwards. It will help to bring your left hand adjacent to your right and push down with that, too. The idea is to try to ease your stomach downwards so it pops out of the hole in the diaphragm. You'll find it easier to do this if an expert shows you first. Some doctors and masseurs may know how. If you can't seem to manage it, try massaging your abdomen with downward movements using your fingertips.

▶ **Long-term programme:**
▶ Surgery might be required. Unfortunately, there's no guarantee that the hiatus hernia won't return.

Irritable bowel syndrome (IBS)

Irritable bowel syndrome (IBS) probably affects about a fifth of Westerners at some time in their lives. Symptoms range from mild to severe. Those symptoms include pain (which in some instances has been likened to giving birth), diarrhoea and/or constipation, bloating and flatulence.

A syndrome is a collection of symptoms and it seems likely that as more is discovered about IBS it will become recognized as several different conditions, with similar symptoms, rather than just one.

▶ **Fast fix:**

▶ Enteric-coated peppermint capsules will relax smooth muscles in the intestines (the coating prevents them dissolving until they get there). But peppermint isn't a long-term solution as (despite the coating) it can also relax the valve between the oesophagus and the stomach, causing heartburn. If you're taking other medications, check with your doctor before taking peppermint capsules.

▶ A hot water bottle on the abdomen may relax the digestive tract and bring some comfort (Chapter 7).

▶ **Long-term programme:**

▶ What's particularly significant is that a high proportion of IBS sufferers were abused as children. If you know you were, or suspect you were, pay particular attention to Chapters 3 and 4.

▶ Self-hypnosis can help you relax your abdominal muscles (Chapter 4).

▶ Some cases can be treated through a diet low in insoluble fibre but high in soluble fibre. Much of the general advice given in Chapter 5 applies. Eat plenty of brown rice, oats, vegetables, peas, beans and lentils (unless any of them are triggers in your case – see below). Avoid fat and oils, including vegetable oils, which can provoke violent intestinal movements in IBS sufferers. This means cutting out/down on fried foods, meat (including poultry) and fish. You may do better with four to five small meals rather than three large ones but don't snack all through the day because there's evidence that the small intestine needs a little free time to do the housework. Certain people are susceptible to specific foods. Common culprits are:

▷ Dairy products

▷ Wheat

▷ Coffee and tea

- ▷ Raw fruits

- ▷ Raw vegetables

- ▷ Beans and bean products.

▶ Learn to relax (Chapter 6).

▶ Take exercise (Chapter 8). A Swedish study of 102 IBS patients, published in 2011, found that those encouraged to take moderate to vigorous exercise for 20 to 30 minutes, three to five times a week, saw a 51 point improvement in their symptoms, compared with a control group of non-exercisers who averaged only a 5 point improvement.

▶ Many IBS sufferers are found to have small intestinal bacterial overgrowth (SIBO). If that's your case it can be cleared up by antibiotics.

▶ Laughter always helps (Chapter 9).

Night cramp

Cramps in the night can be truly agonizing. They most commonly occur in the calf muscles.

▶ **Fast fix:**

▶ Quinine is highly effective at preventing cramps and a tiny quantity is enough. Drinking a glass of quinine-flavoured tonic water at bedtime should do the trick. (Quinine tablets or capsules are not recommended because of their side effects.)

▶ **Long-term programme:**

▶ The cramps occur when the calf muscles are shortened. And they shorten in the night when, unconsciously, you give your legs a stretch and, at the same time, point your toes. By learning not to point your toes you stop the cramps.

▶ Here's what to do. In the daytime practise stretching your legs with your feet and toes turned towards your knees, that's to say, the opposite of pointing your toes. Keep doing it at intervals over several days until it becomes completely automatic. Then whenever you stretch out your legs in your sleep at night your feet and toes will turn back towards your knees without you having to think about it. That will cure it.

▶ If a calf cramp does come on, immediately go into the routine. If you do it quickly enough the pain will stop in a few seconds.

Osteoarthritis (OA)

Unlike rheumatoid arthritis (RA – see below), osteoarthritis (OA) is all about mechanical damage to joints, especially the knees and hips. Whereas RA can start at any age, osteoarthritis is a problem of old age and progresses slowly. It generally affects the hands, hips and knees, specifically through the deterioration of cartilage which normally acts as a cushion. As a result bone rubs on bone in the joint, causing stiffness and pain.

▶ **Fast fix:**

▶ Painkillers, corticosteroid injections, hyaluronic injections, topical capsaicin cream (all in Chapter 2).

▶ **Long-term programme:**

▶ Exercise can extend the range of motion in your joints and develop the muscles that support them (Chapter 8) – walking, cycling and swimming are all good.

▶ Cut down on inflammatory foods and increase your intake of anti-inflammatory foods (Chapter 5).

▶ Vitamin E capsules – 400 IU per day (but 100 IU if you suffer from high blood pressure).

▶ Eat healthily (Chapter 5) to keep your weight down and reduce the strain on your joints – every 10 pounds of excess weight increases the risk of arthritis of the knees by 30 per cent. It's possible that the increased oestrogen produced by fat cells also plays a role.

▶ Acupuncture has proven beneficial in some cases (Chapter 7).

- Laughter always helps (Chapter 9).

- Eventually you may need joint replacement surgery.

Peripheral neuropathy

Peripheral neuropathy, or damage to the peripheral nerves, can be caused by a variety of diseases and in about 30 per cent of cases the cause is unknown (idiopathic). It usually begins with the hands and feet and, as it progresses, sufferers may find their balance affected and have difficulty walking. In some cases sufferers may need to use a wheelchair and in the worst cases it can be fatal. Pain is variable and can be severe. Often there is a burning sensation.

Fast fix:
- Anticonvulsants, antidepressants, local anaesthetics and, for breakthrough pain, opioids (Chapter 2).

Long-term programme:
- Mind Controlled Analgesia (Chapters 3 and 4)

- Alpha-lipoic acid (Chapter 5)

- Capsaicin creams (Chapter 5)

- Stress reduction (Chapter 6)

- Acupuncture (Chapter 7)

- Laughter always helps (Chapter 9)

- TENS (Chapter 10)

Rheumatoid arthritis (RA)

Rheumatoid arthritis (RA) is a dreadful disease in which the body's immune system attacks the body's own cells. It typically begins with the joints of the hands, wrists and feet and the onset is rapid. But RA is about more than joint pain and stiffness. Unlike osteoarthritis (see above), RA sufferers also feel fatigued and ill.

► Fast fix:

► Nonsteroidal anti-inflammatory drugs (NSAIDs), corticosteroids and topical creams (Chapter 2) will reduce the pain.

► Long-term programme:

► The Adverse Childhood Experiences Study involving 15,000 adults in the USA concluded that trauma in early childhood increased the likelihood of autoimmune diseases later in life, notably fibromyalgia, but also including RA. The psychological techniques in Chapters 3 and 4, especially those for tension myositis syndrome (TMS) may help. If you know or suspect that you suffered trauma such as sexual abuse when you were little you may well benefit from professional help.

► Feelings of bitterness, frustration and anger can make RA worse – use the techniques in Chapters 3 and 4 to preserve your tranquillity.

► Emotional upsets can cause RA flare-ups – again the techniques in Chapters 3 and 4 will help.

► Food sensitivities can exacerbate and even cause RA. Eliminate possible triggers from your diet and eat more of the foods that combat inflammation (Chapter 5).

► Eat healthily to keep your weight down and thus reduce the load on your joints (Chapter 5).

► Use relaxation techniques to keep stress at bay (Chapter 6).

► Switch on an electric blanket as soon as you wake up – the warmth will help alleviate the stiffness in your joints (Chapter 7).

► Exercise can help by strengthening the muscles that support the joints as well as by improving stamina (Chapter 8) but keep it light – always pace yourself so, whatever you're doing, you don't get overtired.

► Laughter always helps (Chapter 9).

► TENS is worth a go (Chapter 10).

Key idea

Researchers at the Harvard Medical School followed 100,000 women from 1976 onwards and concluded that those living in the sunniest parts of the USA were 21 per cent less likely to develop RA than those in the cloudiest parts. It's speculated that vitamin D, made by the action of sunlight on the skin, is somehow protective. However, there's no evidence as yet that vitamin D is an effective treatment for RA.

Bibliography

Books

Bales, P. (2008). *Osteoarthritis: Preventing and Healing Without Drugs*. New York: Prometheus Books.

Barnard, N. (1999). *Foods That Fight Pain*. London: Bantam.

Barnard, N. (2010). *The Reverse Diabetes Diet*. Emmaus: Rodale.

Bennett, M. (2010). *Neuropathic Pain*. Oxford: Oxford University Press.

Davies, C. (2004). *The Trigger Point Therapy Workbook*. Oakland: New Harbinger Publications.

Holford. P. (2006). *Say No To Arthritis*. London: Piatkus.

Jenkins, J. (2011). *Rheumatoid Arthritis*. Oxford: How To Books.

Jenner, C. (2011). *Fibromyalgia and Myofascial Pain Syndrome*. Oxford: How To Books.

Key, S. (2000). *Sarah Key's Back Sufferers' Bible*. London: Vermilion.

Lewis, J. (1998). *The Migraine Handbook*. London: Vermilion.

Melzack, R. and Wall, P. D. (1996). *The Challenge of Pain*. London: Penguin.

Rossi, E. L. (1986). *The PsychoBiology Of Mind-Body Healing*. London and New York: Norton.

Sacks, O. (2012). *Migraine*. London: Picador.

Sarno, J. E. (1998). *The Mindbody Prescription*. New York: Warner Books.

Websites

Alexander Technique: www.alexandertechnique.com

American Massage Therapy Association (AMTA): www.amtamassage.org

Arthritis Care: www.arthritiscare.org.uk

British Pain Society: www.britishpainsociety.org

Fibromyalgia Association UK: www.fibromyalgia-associationuk.org

Fibromyalgia network: www.ukfibromyalgia.com

General Council for Massage Therapies, the umbrella body for massage organizations in the UK: www.gcmt.org.uk

Hospice, a site for patients and families facing the pain of a life-threatening illness: www.hospicenet.org

Laughter Yoga International, the website of Dr Madhuri Kataria, the 'inventor' of laughter yoga: www.laughteryoga.org

Migraine Trust: www.migrainetrust.org

National Institute of Neurological Disorders and Stroke: www.ninds.nih.gov/index.htm

Neurology, the journal of the American Academy of Neurology: www.neurology.org

NHS Choices provides all kinds of information and advice from Britain's National Health Service: www.nhs.uk

Pain Concern provides information and support for those in pain: www.painconcern.org.uk

Paul Jenner, author of this book: www.pauljenner.eu

Stanford School of Medicine Pain Management Center: http://paincenter.stanford.edu/

UK Fibromyalgia: www.ukfibromyalgia.com

Index

 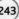